Globalization and Global Health

Understanding Public Health Series

Series editors: Nicki Thorogood and Rosalind Plowman, London School of Hygiene & Tropical Medicine

Understanding Public Health is an innovative series published by Open University Press in collaboration with the London School of Hygiene & Tropical Medicine, where it is used as a key learning resource for postgraduate programmes. It provides self-directed learning covering the major issues in public health affecting low, middle and high income countries.

Titles in the series

Globalization and Global Health

Critical Issues and Policy

Third edition

Edited by Carolyn Stephens, Benjamin Hawkins
and Marco Liverani

 Open University Press

Open University Press
McGraw-Hill Education
8th Floor, 338 Euston Road
London
England
NW1 3BH

email: enquiries@openup.co.uk
world wide web: www.openup.co.uk

and Two Penn Plaza, New York, NY 10121-2289, USA

First edition published 2022

A catalogue record of this book is available from the British Library

Commissioning Editor: Sam Crowe
Associate Editor: Beth Summers
Content Product Manager: Ali Davis
Head of Portfolio Marketing: Bryony Waters

ISBN-13: 9780335249190
ISBN-10: 0335249191
eISBN: 9780335249206

Library of Congress Cataloging-in-Publication Data
CIP data applied for

Typeset by Transforma Pvt. Ltd., Chennai, India
Printed and bound by CPI Group (UK) Ltd, Croydon, CR0 4YY

Praise page

"'Globalization and Global Health' is a unique collection of essays offering a valuable and highly relevant perspective on the relationships between globalization, global health and governances. This book, which is based on a rich and diverse empirical case-studies, highlights the importance of understanding global health as a multi-disciplinary field. Importantly, the book is published in a (post) Covid era and provides important lessons on governance and policy intervention in the field of public health. Pedagogically this book is well structured and is a must-read as in offers a productive lens to understand urgent global health challenges that cross global south/global north division."

Haim Yacobi, Professor of Development Planning and Programme Leader MSc Health in Urban Development at the Bartlett Development Planning Unit, UCL, UK

"This book provides critical issues and policy related to globalization and global health. This book is relevant for everyone that would like to have an overview of current issues of global health in the context of the globalization era. The reflection activities help the readers to digest the book to have comprehensive knowledge."

Ari Probandari, Professor of Public Health at Universitas Sebelas Maret, Indonesia

"I can easily see this book being the 'go-to' text for students of global health. It provides a comprehensive overview of globalisation's impact on health and wellbeing. Crucially, the book also explains the relevance of globalization to the distribution of power across society, and how it has shaped the political and economic determinants of health. With the help of this book, we can hope to see a more critical and politically astute future cohort of global health researchers and practitioners of global health."

Professor David McCoy, United Nations University - International Institute for Global Health, Kuala Lumpur, Malaysia. Formerly Professor of Global Public Health and Director of Education of the Institute of Population Health Sciences, Queen Mary University, London, UK

"This is a very insightful and thought-provoking book on a wide range of issues around globalization and health. It is very timely considering the current challenges the world is facing in this area. It is wide ranging in scope and is up to date in terms of the Covid-19 pandemic that we have

been tackling in recent times. I would recommend this book to anyone with an interest in globalisation and health."

Maggie Wood DNSc, MA in Health Promotion, MSc in Nursing. Department of Nursing, Health Science and Social Care, School of Health Science, Wellbeing and Society, Galway-Mayo Institute of Technology, Ireland

"The importance of Global health policies at the micro and macro levels particularly in developing economies cannot be easily overlooked. Issues of Globalization and Global health are currently on the front burners of health discussion and research in Nigeria vis-à-vis the current Covid-19 pandemic that came as a wake-up call. Currently, there is little or no evidence of Global Health and Global Health Policy as an independent teaching module in our school and I sincerely believe that this book will make a fine contribution towards filling this training gap of our MSc and PhD students at Novena University in particular, and indeed, other Nigerian Universities in general."

Professor Charles C. Ofili, Provost, College of Medical and Health Sciences, Novena University Ogume, Nigeria

"The contributors bring varied expertise to this textbook from a range of interdisciplinary backgrounds, hence making it attractive to a diverse audience, including undergraduate and postgraduate students in the Sciences, Arts and Humanities. Each section clearly guides the reader through three main Global Health areas: Part 1 Contextualising Global Health, Part 2 Critical Issues in Global Health and Part 3 Global Health Governance. Furthermore, each chapter offers structured Learning Objectives, clearly defined Key Terms, focused Activities and Feedback. Overall, the aforementioned makes this a contemporary user-friendly read."

Ms Sarah Jane Renton, Lecturer in Nursing Studies

"For us in the Global South, globalization has influenced and affected several dimensions of life, intensifying historical processes of dependence (not only economic), of exclusion, social inequalities and inequities in health. As the Brazilian Geographer Milton Santos would say, a true fable. In this book, we find not only an important update on a necessary discussion on this topic — and its impacts on health and global governance, but a critical perspective that invites the reader not only to understand theoretical questions, but also to establish dialogues and perspectives that will allow —in the short term, we hope — to decolonize their minds."

Yeimi Alexandra Alzate López. Anthropologist, PhD in Public Health. Institute of Collective Health - Federal University of Bahia, Brazil.

Contents

Conclusions

List of figures, tables, and boxes

Figures

Tables

Boxes

List of contributors

Dr Donald Brown is a Lecturer in Urban Environmental Planning and Governance in the Bartlett Development Planning Unit, University College London.

Dr Benjamin Hawkins is Senior Research Associate in the MRC Epidemiology Unit, University of Cambridge. His research focuses on multi-level governance and corporate political influence in the domain of health policy.

Dr Chris Holden is Reader in International Social Policy in the Department of Social Policy and Social Work, University of York.

Dr Marco Liverani is Associate Professor of Health Policy and Systems in the Department of Global Health and Development, London School of Hygiene & Tropical Medicine. He holds a joint appointment with the School of Tropical Medicine and Global Health, Nagasaki University, and is Honorary Adjunct Professor in the Faculty of Public Health, Mahidol University, in Bangkok.

Aloisia Katsande is a PhD candidate at the London School of Hygiene and Tropical Medicine, working on dietary practices and non-communicable diseases in rural Zimbabwe. Aloisia is also a public health evidence review specialist for a local government in the UK.

Dr Neil Spicer is an Associate Professor in Global Health Policy at the Department of Global Health and Development, London School of Hygiene & Tropical Medicine.

Dr Carolyn Stephens is Honorary Professor of Global Public and Urban Public Health in the Bartlett Development Planning Unit, University College London. She also holds joint appointments with the London School of Hygiene & Tropical Medicine, and University of Tucuman, Argentina. She is an international environmental health and policy specialist, and Module Organizer of the LSHTM elective modules of Globalization and Health, for both the in-house and distance learning MSc programme.

Dr Preslava Stoeva is an Assistant Professor at the Department of Global Health and Development, London School of Hygiene & Tropical Medicine, where she is Course Director of the MSc Global Health Policy (DL).

Acknowledgements

Open University Press and the London School of Hygiene & Tropical Medicine have made every effort to obtain permission from copyright holders to reproduce material in this book and to acknowledge these sources correctly. Any omissions brought to our attention will be remedied in future editions.

We would like to express our grateful thanks to the copyright holders for granting permission to reproduce material in this book from the following sources:

Wellcome Trust: Actual and supposed routes of cholera from Hindoostan to Europe and North America in 1832, 1848, 1854, 1867 and 1873, from *A Treatise on Asiatic Cholera*, edited and prepared by Edmund Charles Wendt in association with John C. Peters, 1885. © Wellcome Collection. Attribution 4.0 International (CC BY 4.0). **(Figure 5.1)**

World Health Organization: Decision instrument for the assessment and notification of events that may constitute a public health emergency of international concern in the IHR 2005. **(Figure 5 3)**

United Nations Environment Programme: Relationships between human populations and their economic and social activities, and the resultant links of the ecosystem with human health and activities **(Figure 7.1)**

Introduction to globalization and health

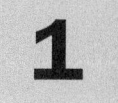

Benjamin Hawkins, Carolyn Stephens and Marco Liverani

Overview

This chapter provides an introduction to the concepts of globalization, global health and global health governance that underpin the issues discussed in this volume. It begins by discussing the highly contested term 'globalization'. It sets out a conceptual framework for understanding the distinct features of globalization and attempts to place current forms of globalization within their historical context as the consequence of specific technological and political developments. It links the closely related concepts of governance and global governance to the specific issues of global health and global health governance. The chapter concludes with an overview of the book, the key issues and topics addressed.

Learning objectives

After working through this chapter, you will be able to:

- Define and critique the concepts of globalization, governance and global health governance.
- Apply a conceptual framework for understanding globalization and its links with historical and contemporary developments in global health.
- Understand the ways in which processes of globalization are of relevance for current issues and debates in global health.

Key terms

Globalization: A set of processes, facilitated by technological developments, leading to greater economic, political, cultural and environmental interconnectedness across the globe.

Global health: A field of research, scholarship, policy and practice focused on health issues where the determinants or outcomes are not contained by the territorial boundaries of states, and thus may be beyond the capacity of individual countries to address them through domestic institutions alone.

Governance: A series of arrangements consisting of various norms, rules and institutional structures through which an area of economic activity, public policy or social interaction is regulated and administered by a range of public and private actors.

Global health governance: The shifting array of institutions, structures, mechanisms and actors through which issues in the arena of global health are identified and addressed and through which policy responses are decided and implemented.

Imperialism: A policy of extending a country's power and influence through diplomacy, political power, trade or military force: for example, Western imperialism. Anti-imperialism describes the movement against this.

Neo-liberalism: This term refers generally to processes that include the reduction of state power: state interventions are minimized; privatization, finance and market processes are emphasized; capital controls and trade restrictions are eased; free markets, free trade and free enterprise are summary terms for this process.

What is globalization?

The concept of 'globalization' is often described as a set of political, social and institutional processes that have occurred since the early 1980s, driven by economic change and increasing market liberalization across borders. However, the term globalization is highly contested, and its precise meaning is a source of constant debate. There is disagreement about whether globalization is actually happening, or at least whether it is happening in uniform and consistent ways across the globe, and if it is concentrated in particular geographical locations and sectors of policy and the economy. Similarly, there are debates about whether the processes we have observed in recent decades represent something fundamentally new and qualitatively different from events and processes in previous eras. Certainly, technological developments in recent decades, particularly the creation of the internet and information technology, have affected the nature of global interconnection and interdependence as discussed below. Yet the nineteenth and early twentieth centuries saw high levels of international trade within the context of European imperialism, and the term globalization itself has been in use since the 1930s (James and Steger 2014).

Recent debates have centred on whether the phase of globalization that we date back to the 1980s continues today, or whether we have entered a new phase of stasis or even partial retrenchment in the movement towards global interconnection and interdependence. Events since the mid-2010s have seen at least a rhetorical rejection of the ideal of globalization, and the 'globalist' values that underpin it, from some political actors and a re-emphasizing of the nation state as the most important legitimate political community.

Debates about globalization are inextricably linked to those about power and global justice. The specific forms that globalization has taken since the 1980s at least – and arguably since the end of the Second World War – often reflect the interests of the most powerful states and economic actors. This includes the political and institutional structures established by high-income countries, including the United Nations, whose leadership roles and, to a great extent, activities, continue to be dominated by these high-income countries. From this perspective, globalization is often criticized as a form of neo-colonialism through which transnational businesses and their client governments extract value and resources from low- and middle-income countries (LMICs) through unfair and exploitative practices, many of which are historically entrenched in the global system (Wallerstein 1974; Bhambra 2021). Before we examine these issues, which are addressed throughout the book, it is first important to explore and unpack the concept of globalization. In the following sections, we set out a framework for understanding globalization.

Scholars in many disciplines have attempted to define the concept of globalization. Most agree that it is a process that involves increasing interconnection across multiple spheres of activity between regions, countries and individuals. Globalization has a range of social, economic, environmental and health *impacts* that are increasingly felt by people across the globe, including infectious and non-communicable disease patterns. Here are some examples of how globalization has been defined:

a stretching of social, political and economic activities across frontiers such that events, decisions and activities in one region of the world can come to have significance for individuals and communities in distant regions of the globe. (Held et al. 1999)

what we in the Third World have for several centuries called colonization. (Khor 1995)

the intensification of worldwide social relations which link distant localities in such a way that local happenings are shaped by events occurring many miles away and vice-versa. (Giddens 1990)

In a general sense, the increasing worldwide integration of economic, cultural, political, religious, and social systems. Economic globalization is the process by which the whole world becomes a single market. This means that goods and services, capital, and labour are traded on a world-wide basis, and information and the results of research flow readily between countries. (Oxford Reference 2021)

the increase of trade around the world, especially by large companies producing and trading goods in many different countries . . . a situation in which available goods and services, or social and cultural influences, gradually become similar in all parts of the world. (Cambridge Dictionary 2021)

Activity 1.1

Reflect on the definitions of globalization above. Which of these definitions do you find most useful? Have you seen them used and discussed in relation to (global) health policy? If so, in which contexts and in relation to which specific issues?

Feedback

As you can see, there are many different definitions of globalization. You may prefer a definition that emphasizes the social aspects of these processes, or one that focuses on the trade and economic aspects. Having settled on your preferred definition, perhaps you tried to apply it to your own context. If you have seen these definitions applied in the context of health policy, maybe that was in relation to trade in health services or specific aspects of health policy, such as access to medicines and the Doha Declaration. For each of these definitions, think through their implications for health policy and health.

Conceptualizing globalization

One way of thinking about and examining processes of globalization is to look at the key characteristics of the changes that these processes encompass. For example, Lee (2003) has developed an analytical framework for examining globalization in terms of its spatial, temporal and cognitive dimensions.

The spatial dimension

A key aspect of globalization is the fundamental shift in the way in which human beings interact with territorial space. Large parts of the global population are now mobile in ways that would have been unimaginable even one or two generations ago. Historically, travel was expensive, time-consuming and, where possible at all, was limited to very short distances and small sections of the population. Since the 1980s, however, it has become increasingly affordable for large sections of the population, at least in high- and middle-income countries, to travel more frequently and over much longer distances for work and pleasure.

In the past decades there has been an unprecedented increase in human mobility. In 2019, the number of international migrants globally reached an estimated 272 million, accounting for 3.5 per cent of the world population. This was 119 million more than in 1990 and over three times the estimated number in 1970 (International Organization for Migration 2020). By the end of 2018, there was a total of 25.9 million refugees globally – the highest number on record (UNHCR 2019). Tourism has also increased exponentially, becoming one of the world's most important economic activities since its origins in Western Europe in the seventeenth century. In recent decades, it has grown rapidly due to technological and regulatory innovations, which brought greater comfort, speed and lower cost to travel. In 2019, according to official data of the World Tourism Organization, international tourist arrivals worldwide grew by 4 per cent to reach 1.5 billion (UN World Tourism Organization 2020).

In many ways, increasing population mobility is a positive trend, which can contribute to socio-economic development, welfare, and cultural diversity and understanding, both in the countries visited by tourists and in the countries receiving refugees. However, with this movement of peoples globally come important implications for global health. As people and goods move around the world, they can spread microbes and pathogens from one location to another. This was how the Covid-19 pandemic was able to spread so rapidly around the world after its initial identification in Wuhan, China, in late 2019. Similarly, the movement of health workers and patients across borders brings additional challenges discussed below.

The temporal dimension

This aspect of globalization relates to the ways in which we perceive and experience time and is closely connected to the spatial component described above. With technological innovations we are able to move more quickly and across greater distances, and communicate immediately with all parts of the world via online platforms. As the economic geographer David Harvey argued, this 'time-space compression' is a fundamental driver of globalization, characterized by the intensification of events and interactions across wider spaces and in shorter times (Harvey 1992). Harvey was particularly concerned with the global flow of capital, which moves at ever-increasing speeds thanks to advances in information technology. Similarly, the remittance economy has grown enormously through online remittance providers, reaching a record US$689 billion in 2018, including US$528 billion to LMICs (World Bank 2019). These changes have also affected the arena of global health through, for example, the development of remote health service provision (e-medicine), enhanced research collaborations and policy networks between actors across the globe.

The cognitive dimension

The cognitive dimension refers to how globalization is changing the ways in which we perceive the world as a result of these technological developments (see Chapter 3). The advent of the internet and new forms of media and information exchange, including a constantly evolving range of social media platforms, have revolutionized the ways in which information is created, exchanged and consumed. Until the 1980s, media remained largely national in scope. The markets were constrained by both political/regulatory boundaries (e.g. laws about foreign media ownership) as well as linguistic ones. Since then, however, there has been a move towards transnational ownership of the media with the emergence of large multinational media conglomerates. In addition, the impact of the internet on modes of communications has led to the emergence of an increasingly global 'online' public sphere. This has come to be dominated by a small number of global media behemoths with enormous power to shape the information we are able to access and, with this, the norms and values that inform political discourse (Machin and Van Leeuwen 2007; Shirky 2011). Thus, online communication has provided an unprecedented outlet for millions of people to express their views, feelings and ideas. At the same time, corporations and political actors can use their power to filter that information. The rise of social media has also seen a proliferation of 'fake news' and misinformation, with important implications for health and healthcare. During the Covid-19 pandemic, for example, there was a wave of misinformation about miracle therapies, the extent of the pandemic and the clinical effects of vaccines, not backed by reliable evidence. In light of this, the WHO and other UN agencies issued official statements urging governments to fight what they called 'infodemic' or information epidemics (WHO et al. 2020).

Challenging globalization

For much of the period since the late 1980s, globalization was often identified as a permanent global force with a clear and unidirectional vector of travel. This led to a perception that the international system of nation states was gradually morphing into a global web of interdependencies, which challenged long-standing notions of national sovereignty (Marsh et al. 2006). Proponents of processes of globalization argue that the course of history involves the decline of the state and of territoriality as a viable form of political organization or meaningful unit of analysis for understanding social and political change. They suggest that political power is situated in new global configurations and processes, expressed through transnational actors (such as global corporations) and institutions rather than states (Steger 2020). In other words, it was, and often is, assumed that the direction of travel is necessarily towards a 'borderless world', characterized by ever greater cross-border interactions and interdependence.

Since the early 1990s, we have seen a range of critiques of the modern forms of globalization – sometimes 'anti-globalist', often articulated as opposition to corporate power (Eschle 2004), sometimes arguing for 'glocalization' (Khondker 2005). The latter concept is perhaps particularly resonant in countries trying to protect their cultural history in the face of powerful global actors promoting a homogenizing message. Bishop and Payne (2021) argue that 'globalization remains contested, and often misunderstood, with damaging real-world consequences', and that it is a complex process that is here to stay. They argue that it is often the particular form which current patterns of globalization have taken – 'neo-liberal' social and political forces controlled by powerful actors – which is the issue and should be reformed and re-envisioned.

Some critics of globalization have argued that these modern relationships of interdependence between the Global North and Global South reproduce colonial forms of exploitation through other means (Khor 1995). These concerns were a central part of the emerging anti-globalization movement in the 1990s and early 2000s, including civil society movements protesting against neo-liberalism and corporate power (Eschle 2004). In certain regions during the late 1990s and early 2000s this saw the election of a series of governments opposed to economic globalization. For example, in Central and South America from the early 2000s the presidents of Brazil, Argentina, Ecuador, Venezuela and Bolivia were all elected on similar platforms, which became known as the Pink Tide, opposing economic neo-liberalism and the proliferation of free trade agreements that favoured expansion of global corporations in the region (Castañeda 2006; Nilsson 2012).

It is also notable that a different aspect of 'anti-globalization' emerged in the second decade of the 2000s, with nationalist-populist administrations being elected internationally (Achilles et al. 2018). Where these governments are in powerful countries with global reach, this can have major repercussions globally. For example, the United States (2016) and Brazil (2018) both elected presidents standing on explicitly 'anti-globalist' platforms who then challenged the global consensus on a number of global policy issues, including environmental protection and trade. For example, on entering office in January 2017, US President Donald Trump immediately signalled his intention to withdraw the US from the Trans-Pacific Partnership

Agreement and negotiations on another trade agreement with the EU, the Trans-Atlantic Trade and Investment Agreement (TTIP), were halted. This was followed by decisions to withdraw from other multinational agreements including the Paris Climate Agreement and the Joint Comprehensive Plan of Action on the Iranian nuclear programme. Collectively, this represented a seismic reorientation of US foreign policy and the rejection of multilateral norms and institutions (Debaere 2018). It also illustrates the power of changing popular views of globalization and their potential impact on national and global politics (Achilles et al. 2018; Nilsen 2016).

In the economic sector, it is also notable that the global trade regime has experienced a period of impasse since 2002, following a period of deeper integration in the preceding decades, which culminated with the formation of the World Trade Organization (WTO) in 1995. The WTO provides the basic rules of international trade. The 'Doha Development Round' of WTO trade negotiations stalled soon after its launch in 2001. Consequently, the international trade regime has seen a proliferation of bilateral, regional and trade agreements, including those cited above in the intervening period (see Chapter 13).

The entry of China into the global economy since the 1980s has also influenced and reshaped processes that we know as globalization, not least through the outsourcing of large sectors of global manufacturing from their home countries to China with consequences for the structure of economies across the world. China is now one of the three largest economies in the world (alongside the US and the EU) and is pursuing a policy of global economic (and increasingly also geo-strategic) expansionism. China has invested significantly in sub-Saharan Africa, particularly in the commodity and resources sectors (e.g. oil, copper and nickel) of key strategic value to the industrial and high tech sectors (Ericsson et al. 2020).

Despite the developments noted above, it is not possible to state that the processes of globalization have drawn to a halt or even gone into reverse. Instead, we have arguably entered a new phase of globalization in which the contours of global systems and interconnections have shifted and in which the dynamics of the process are perhaps more complex than in previous eras. This has been called 'reglobalization' (Bishop and Payne 2021). It could be argued that the concept of globalization – with its implicit teleology towards a more global and integrated international system – is no longer the most appropriate term to describe the phenomenon that we are seeking to study. The economic and political systems that are evolving represent an increasingly uneven, non-linear and non-unidirectional form of shifting inter-connection and interdependencies between political and economic actors at and above the level of the nation state, which we can term 'asymmetric globalization'. These asymmetries play themselves out through complex power relationships operating globally.

So far in this section we have seen what could be termed the 'empirical challenge' to globalization from those who question whether globalization – in a truly global sense – has ever occurred or is continuing to occur in the current era. However, globalization is also being challenged in an

increasingly normative sense. The history of the anti-globalization movement dates back almost as far as the existence of the term globalization
itself and the emergence of the political-economic developments that it
describes (Eschle 2004). An example of the anti-globalization movement of
the 1990s was the so-called 'battle of Seattle' in 1999 - in which protests
against the WTO, led by anti-globalization activists and timed to coincide
with the ministerial conference held in the city, led to violent battles
between protesters and local police who deployed water cannons and other
tactics to disperse the crowds. The lessons of this, including for the WTO,
were extensively documented and debated (Kahn and Kellner 2004).

The legacy of the WTO protests, and the enduring impasse in WTO negotiations since the early 2000s, has led the anti-globalization movement to
shift focus onto other forums, including the negotiation of mega-regional
agreements such as the TTIP, which were the subject also of significant
civil society mobilization. The intervening period has also seen the emergence of civil society responses to these processes, both in the North and
the South whose objectives are focused, at least in part, on mitigating the
consequences of globalization (e.g. Harris 2003; Agarwala 2007; Gümrükçü 2010; Nilsen 2016).

The consequences of these historical experiences are clearly obvious in
the field of global health in terms of access to health services and products, while the wider economic and political regimes are structural drivers
of population health and health systems capacity. In many ways, the
debate about globalization links to, and leads from, the debate about the
concept of 'development', which has strong associations with colonialism
by Western powers, and has been debated and critiqued repeatedly (Escobar 1995; Shivji 2002; Nilsen 2016). The search for global justice in the
context of health and beyond thus depends on a questioning and reorgani-
zation of the current global order. This does not necessarily imply an 'end'
to globalization *per se*, if this is even possible, but the promotion of new
forms of globalization that promote a more equitable distribution of
resources and outcomes. This in turn implies the creation of more just and
democratic forms of governance mechanisms to oversee and implement
these emerging structures. We turn to the question of governance in the
following section.

Global governance and health

Alongside globalization, another key concept with which the current book
engages is that of governance. It is easiest to understand the concept of
governance alongside the (perhaps) more established concept of government. The latter refers to formal mechanisms of decision-making which are
closely associated with the state. We often speak about national, regional,
local and municipal governments, which derive their authority and powers
from the state and its constitutional structures. Government implies established institutional structures such as local councils, national parliaments,

ministries and bureaucracies (i.e. civil servants and administrators). Governance, meanwhile, implies a decentring or problematization of the notion of government to include not just new structures and decision-making forums but multiple actors and agencies beyond the state. This includes the involvement of private sector actors, including transnational corporations, and civil society actors such as charities and non-governmental organizations (NGOs).

The UN Commission on Global Governance (1995: 2) defines governance as the formal and informal arrangements through which 'individuals and institutions, public and private, manage their common affairs' and through which 'conflicting or diverse interests may be accommodated, and cooperative action may be taken'. The shift from government to governance has been evident in developments at the national level as state governments have increasingly 'outsourced' policy implementation and even policymaking capacity to autonomous or semi-autonomous bodies and agencies. This includes the creation of public–private partnership, self-government and co-regulatory arrangements involving the private sector (i.e. corporations and businesses). However, it is perhaps at the global level that this shift has been most obvious and had the most impact.

As we shall see in Chapter 9, there is no equivalent of national governments above the level of the state. There is no 'world government', so policymaking and implementation at the global level occurs in different ways to that at the national level. Because of the prevailing conditions in the global system, decision-making and implementation at the global level often fall under the rubric of governance. The term 'global governance' has entered the lexicon of scholars seeking to examine these processes. Governance arrangements at the global level often involve multiple actors debating and responding to issues in a variety of (sometimes) parallel and overlapping forums and structures. For example, perceived failures of the World Health Organization (WHO) response to HIV/AIDS led to the formation of a new agency, UNAIDS, under the auspices of another branch of the United Nations (UN) system (see Chapter 10). In addition, recent decades have seen a proliferation of new types of actors engaged in the arena of global governance (see Chapters 11, 12 and 14).

These developments have been particularly evident in the area of global health - including private philanthropic bodies (e.g. the Bill and Melinda Gates Foundation) and public–private partnerships (e.g. the Global Fund) (see Chapter 12). It has led to the emergence of a global heath governance as a distinct area of political activity and scholarly analysis. Fidler (2010: 3) defines global health governance as 'the use of formal and informal institutions, rules, and processes by states, intergovernmental organizations, and nonstate actors to deal with challenges to health that require cross-border collective action to address effectively' (see also Chapters 4 and 12). It is these institutions, rules, actors, challenges and outcomes in different areas of health policy that are the focus of the chapters in the book.

Activity 1.2

In light of the discussion above - reflect on the relevance of processes of globalization for global health. What are the key ways in which globalization impacts on determinants of global health and health itself?

Feedback

In your answer you may have considered some of the following issues. Globalization leads to increasing movements of people, animals and goods across borders, which may lead to increasing movement of pathogens with the consequence of infectious disease outbreaks. This requires global, coordinated policy responses at the level of international organizations and mechanisms.

Trade in food, alcohol and other commodities, and the entry of transnational businesses which sell them, into new markets may lead to changes in diet and lifestyle which, allied with technological advances, may have implications for population health, obesity and related non-communicable diseases.

Increasing exchanges of information across borders, however, has the possibility to increases global awareness of health issues and to build movements and political pressure to address these through both traditional and innovative policy mechanisms.

Globalization is linked to global environmental changes through increased consumption and waste. This includes climate change, loss of biodiversity, waste, destruction of food and water essential ecosystems. There are multiple health outcomes associated with these changes.

There are many other links you may have thought of.

Overview of the book

This book is organized into sections. This introduction starts the textbook. It is followed by three parts: Part 1 Contextualizing global health; Part 2 Critical issues in global health; and Part 3 Global health governance. The book then concludes with a chapter on trends in the theme of globalization and health over time and reflections on overall themes.

Chapter 1 looks at the concept of globalization and its links to health. It looks at trends in global health research over time. It also introduces the structure of the book and outlines how the book is organized.

Part 1 attempts to place current issues and developments in global health in their economic, social and historical context. Chapter 2 presents an overview of the structure of, and key developments in, the global economy, placing debates in global health within the wider economic context. Chapter 3 complements this by examining the major changes in social conditions in recent decades and their implications for global health, including the historical colonial heritage of global social trends and emergence of social media and other transformative technologies. Chapter 4 then offers a historical overview of global health governance from its origins to the present day, identifying the colonial origins of global public health and the repercussions of this through to the current era.

Part 2 offers an overview of the key issues in global health. Chapter 5 discusses infectious diseases as an enduring issue in global health, often rooted in colonial approaches to disease control, while Chapter 6 charts the emergence of non-communicable diseases as a truly global health challenge. Both chapters explore the effects of these trends internationally. Chapter 7 discusses global environmental changes as a key structural determinant of health, while Chapter 8 discusses the increasing tendency to treat global health issues as a security challenge and the consequences of this securitization.

Part 3 focuses on key actors and institutions in global health governance. Chapter 9 analyses the changing role of the state as an actor in global health governance, highlighting the enduring importance of states despite the limitations to their powers in the global sphere and the emergence of other important global health actors. Chapter 10 examines the bilateral and multilateral structures and mechanisms (such as international organizations like WHO) through which global health governance occurs. Chapter 11 discusses the role of the commercial sector and, in particular, transnational corporations as 'commercial determinants' of health and as key actors within global health governance. The focus of Chapter 12 is on global civil society actors and non-governmental actors in global health, contrasting these organizations to those in the commercial sector discussed in the preceding chapter. Chapter 13 examines the global trade regime and the relevance of cross-border trade in goods and services for global health, including the use of international trade and investment agreements to challenge health policies.

Chapter 14 draws together the key themes and insights from the book and seeks to link these to the emerging trends and dynamics in global health. It adopts a critical stance towards the discipline of global health and reflects the discussion in Chapter 4 of the colonial heritage of the discipline. It then reflects on shifts in understanding since the first edition of this textbook and ways that these debates may shape future development in global health and global health governance.

Summary

This chapter introduced the theme of globalization and health and discussed the highly contested concept of globalization. Having set out some of the key definitions used in the scholarly literature, we presented a simple conceptual framework through which to analyse processes of globalization and their relevance for global health. The chapter then introduced the concepts of global health and global governance that will be explored throughout the book. Finally, it introduced the structure of the book and the key focus of each of the following chapters.

References

Achilles, M., Kunakhovich, K. and Shea, N. (2018) Nationalism, nativism, and the revolt against globalization, *Europe Now*. Available at: https://globalization.europenowjournal.org/2018/01/31/nationalism-nativism-and-the-revolt-against-globalization/ (accessed 21 June 2021).

Agarwala, R. (2007) Resistance and compliance in the age of globalization: Indian women and labor organizations, *Annals of the American Academy of Political and Social Science*, 610: 143–159.

Bhambra, G.K. (2021) Colonial global economy: towards a theoretical reorientation of political economy, *Review of International Political Economy*, 28(2): 307–322.

Bishop, M. and Payne, A. (2021) The political economies of different globalizations: theorizing reglobalization, *Globalizations*, 18(1): 1–21.

Cambridge Dictionary (2021) Globalization definition. Available at: https://dictionary.cambridge.org/dictionary/english/globalization (accessed 21 June 2021).

Castañeda, J.G. (2006) Latin America's left turn, *Foreign Affairs*, 85(3): 28–43.

Commission on Global Governance (1995) *Our Global Neighbourhood*. Oxford: Oxford University Press.

Debaere, P. (2018) Globalization under fire, *Europe Now*. Available at: https://globalization.europenowjournal.org/2018/01/31/globalization-under-fire/ (accessed 21 June 2021).

Ericsson, M., Löf, O. and Löf, A. (2020) Chinese control over African and global mining – past, present and future, *Mineral Economics*, 33: 153–181.

Eschle, C. (2004) Constructing 'the anti-globalization movement', *International Journal of Peace Studies*, 9(1): 61–84.

Escobar, A. (1995) *Encountering Development: The Making and Unmaking of the Third World*. Princeton, NJ: Princeton University Press.

Fidler, D. (2010) *The Challenges of Global Health Governance*. New York: Council on Foreign Relations.

Giddens, A. (1990) *The Consequences of Modernity*. Stanford, CA: Stanford University Press.

Gümrükçü, S. (2010) The rise of a social movement: the emergence of anti-globalization movements in Turkey, *Turkish Studies*, 11(2): 163–180.

Harris, R. (2003) Popular resistance to globalization and neoliberalism in Latin America, *Journal of Developing Societies*, 19(2–3): 365–426.

Harvey, D. (1992) *The Condition of Postmodernity: An Enquiry into the Origins of Cultural Change*. Oxford: Blackwell Publishers.

Held, D., McGrew, A., Goldblatt, D. et al. (1999) *Global Transformations, Politics, Economics and Culture*. Stanford, CA: Stanford University Press.

International Organization for Migration (2020) *World Migration Report*. Available at: https://publications.iom.int/system/files/pdf/wmr_2020.pdf (accessed 15 June 2021)

James, P. and Steger, M. (2014) A genealogy of 'globalization': the career of a concept, *Globalizations*, 11(4): 417–434.

Kahn, R. and Kellner, D. (2004) New media and internet activism: from the 'Battle of Seattle' to blogging, *New Media & Society*, 6(1): 87–95.

Khondker, H. (2005) Globalization to glocalisation: a conceptual exploration, *Intellectual Discourse*, 13(2): 181–199.

Khor, M. (1995) Globalization and the need for coordinated southern policy response, *Cooperation South, Special Issue*, pp. 15–18. New York: UNDP.

Lee, K. (2003) *Globalization and Health: An Introduction*. London: Palgrave Macmillan.

Machin, D. and Van Leeuwen, T. (2007) *Global Media Discourse: A Critical Introduction*. Abingdon: Routledge.

Marsh, D., Smith, M.J. and Hothi, N. (2006) Globalization and the state, in C. Hay, M. Lister and D. Marsh (eds) *The State: Theories and Issues*. London: Red Globe Press.

Nilsen, A. (2016) Power, resistance and development in the Global South: notes towards a critical research agenda, *International Journal of Politics, Culture and Society*, 29: 269–287.

Nilsson, M. (2012) Globalization and the formation of the political left in Latin America, in M. Nilsson and J. Gustafsson (eds) *Latin American Responses to Globalization in the 21st Century*. London: Palgrave Macmillan.

Oxford Reference (2021) Overview globalization, *Quick Reference*. Available at: https://globalization. oxfordreference.com/view/10.1093/oi/authority.20110803095855259 (accessed 21 June 2021)

Shirky, C. (2011) The political power of social media: technology, the public sphere, and political change, *Foreign Affairs*, 90(1): 28–41.

Shivji, I. (2002) Globalization and popular resistance, in J. Semboja, J. Mwapachu and E. Jansen (eds) *Local Perspectives on Globalization: The African Case*. Dar es Salaam: Mkuki na Nyota Publishers.

Steger, M. (2020) *Globalization: A Very Short Introduction*. Oxford: Oxford University Press.

UN World Tourism Organization (2020) World tourism barometer No. 18: January 2020. Available at: https://globalization.unwto.org/world-tourism-barometer-n18-january-2020 (accessed 16 July 2021).

United Nations High Commissioner for Refugees (UNHCR) (2019) Global trends: forced displacement in 2018. Available at: https://globalization.unhcr.org/5d08d7ee7.pdf (accessed 16 July 2021).

Wallerstein, I. (1974) The rise and future demise of the world capitalist system: concepts for comparative analysis, *Comparative Studies in Society and History*, 16(4): 387–415.

World Bank (2019) *Migration and Remittances: Recent Developments and Outlook. Migration and Development Brief 31*. Washington, DC: The World Bank. Available at: https://globalization.knomad. org/publication/migration-and-development-brief-31 (accessed 16 July 2021).

World Health Organization (WHO) The United Nations (UN), UNICEF et al. (2020) Managing the Covid-19 infodemic: promoting healthy behaviours and mitigating the harm from misinformation and disinformation. Joint statement by WHO, UN, UNICEF, UNDP, UNESCO, UNAIDS, ITU, UN Global Pulse, and IFRC. Available at: https://globalization.who.int/news/item/23-09-2020-managing-the-Covid-19-infodemic-promoting-healthy-behaviours-and-mitigating-the-harm-from-misinformation-and-disinformation (accessed 12 June 2021).

PART 1

Contextualizing global health

Introduction to the global economy

2

Chris Holden

Overview

This chapter will examine the main features of the global economy and how it has changed over time. It will provide an outline of the historical development of the global economy and will introduce international trade, foreign direct investment and financial globalization as the three main components of economic globalization. It will then introduce the most important intergovernmental organizations that provide the framework for global economic governance, specifically the International Monetary Fund, the World Bank and the World Trade Organization. The chapter will also consider the principal impacts of economic globalization on economic growth, poverty and inequality around the world. The chapter relates closely to Chapter 2 and its analysis of social trends; the analysis of bilateral and multilateral actors in Chapter 10, and global trade and health in Chapter 13.

Learning objectives

After working through this chapter you will be able to:

- Understand how the global economy has changed over time.
- Identify the main components of economic globalization.
- Describe how the International Monetary Fund, World Bank and World Trade Organization are organized and their roles in global economic governance.
- Critically assess the impacts of economic globalization on poverty and inequality.

Key terms

Economic globalization: The processes by which goods, services, investment capital and the ownership of financial assets flow across borders and the resulting integration of national economies.

Foreign direct investment: The process of investing in a business operation overseas to produce a good or provide a service.

Financial globalization: The trading of currencies and financial assets across national borders.

Global economic governance: The processes, structures and rules by which intergovernmental organizations and other actors attempt to regulate the global economy.

International trade: The exchange of goods and services between people or entities that reside in different countries.

Introduction

Economic processes are important social determinants of health. How economies work, whether they are growing or not, the level of (un)employment, the quality of working conditions and how income and wealth are distributed all contribute to the physical and mental well-being of billions of people around the globe. One of the most important features of economic life today is economic globalization, that is, the growing integration of national economies, so that we may speak of a 'global economy'. This means that more of what is consumed in any given country is produced in another country than was the case in the past, that the owners of many large businesses in any given country may reside abroad, and that money and ownership entitlements may be transferred between people in different countries in as little as a few minutes. Therefore, key social determinants of health, such as income levels, the ability or otherwise to meet citizens' basic needs, economic security or precarity, working conditions and employment levels are at least partially dependent upon an economy that is global in scope. Where a country is able to harness the forces of the global economy to increase the income and wealth of its people, levels of poverty can be substantially reduced, and governments have more resources that can be used to provide health and other services. However, the distribution of economic gains within and between countries is also crucial in determining outcomes. Moreover, economic crises of the type that occurred in 2007–2009 can spread rapidly around the globe, causing dramatic increases in unemployment and poverty and transforming people's ability to meet their needs.

While economic processes are important social determinants of health, health and health policies can also have important consequences for the performance of economies. Massive falls in economic output resulted from the necessary actions of governments to contain the Covid-19 pandemic that began in early 2020. Less dramatically, the health of a country's people may affect both their ability to work and their productivity. So, health and the global economy are inextricably linked. Furthermore, economic globalization is often connected to other aspects of globalization, such as technological or cultural change (see Chapter 3). Consequently, an understanding of the global economy is necessary for an understanding of globalization more generally.

A brief history of the global economy

To understand the processes of economic globalization, it is helpful to place current trends and institutions within the context of how the global economy has developed over time. While some authors characterize economic globalization as a relatively new phenomenon, dating from the 1980s, others argue that it has been around much longer (Hirst et al. 2009).

Activity 2.1

Consider the following quote, and identify three ways in which it describes the global economy. Consider who might have written this and when:

. . . the world market [has] given a cosmopolitan character to production and consumption in every country . . . it has drawn from under the feet of industry the national ground on which it stood. All old-established national industries have been destroyed or are daily being destroyed. They are dislodged by new industries, whose introduction becomes a life and death question for all civilised nations, by industries that no longer work up indigenous raw material, but raw material drawn from the remotest zones; industries whose products are consumed, not only at home, but in every quarter of the globe. In place of the old wants, satisfied by the production of the country, we find new wants, requiring for their satisfaction the products of distant lands and climes. In place of the old local and national seclusion and self-sufficiency, we have intercourse in every direction, universal interdependence of nations.

Feedback

You might have considered how well (or not) this quote describes our modern globalized economy. You might have identified the discussion of the way that the global economy draws countries into interdependent, competitive relationships. You might have commented on the idea of social change including consumerism, and the rise of the 'new wants' (see Chapter 3 for more on this). You might have considered the discussion of the impact of these new processes on the nation state and its independence.

You might be surprised to know that this was written by Marx and Engels in 1848 (Marx and Engels, 2018: 5). You might now consider whether your analysis of this quote identified any processes that were missing from Marx and Engel's analysis, or that have changed since they wrote this. For example, there is reference here to colonialism, if not named as such. There is also no mention here of the international organizations we have come to regard as permanent features of global governance.

During the latter half of the nineteenth century, trade between the European powers, as well as between the European powers and the USA, grew extensively, albeit with much of the rest of the world tied into the system through coercive, colonial power structures. This early form of economic globalization broke down with the outbreak of the First World War. The period between the world wars was one that might be characterized as 'deglobalization'.

Activity 2.2

Go to the 'Trade and Globalization' pages of the 'Our World in Data' website (https://ourworldindata.org/trade-and-globalization). Scroll down to the section on 'Trade from a historical perspective'. Look to see how trade openness has grown over the last few centuries, and particularly from the nineteenth century onwards. Has the world become more globalized over time by this measure?

Feedback

You should see that trade openness, measured by the ratio of trade (imports plus exports) to gross domestic product (GDP), grew during the final decades of the nineteenth century before declining, and then grew steeply after the Second World War. However, look a little more carefully at the charts and the main text – you should be able to see during which periods of crisis in the twentieth and twenty-first centuries trade declined.

The Wall Street Crash of 1929 saw the New York stock exchange collapse, triggering the Great Depression of the 1930s (Galbraith 2009). The gold standard, the fixed exchange rate system that had been in place for much of the nineteenth century and early twentieth century, was abandoned (exchange rate systems will be discussed in a little more depth in the next section). In the run-up to the Second World War, countries implemented protectionist trade policies and competitive currency devaluation, in vain attempts to boost their own exports and limit imports, resulting in a general decline of trade and economic stagnation.

After the Second World War, the Western Allied powers, under US leadership, resolved to build a more orderly economic governance architecture in order to avoid the mistakes of the inter-war period and cohere the capitalist powers against the perceived threat from the Soviet Union. Old colonial relationships such as the British Empire were dismantled, with colonized countries gaining their independence over time.

Many of the institutions that still play a major role in the governance of the world economy, such as the World Bank and International Monetary Fund (IMF), discussed below, were created at the end of the Second World War. The General Agreement on Tariffs and Trade (GATT) system was created in 1947 to provide a forum in which governments could negotiate with each other to reduce trade barriers. A new, more flexible fixed exchange rate system was introduced, the Bretton Woods monetary system – named after the US town in which the conference establishing the World Bank and IMF was held – where the exchange rates of other major currencies were tied to the US dollar and the value of the dollar was itself tied to gold. The period up to the 1970s saw relative economic stability and rapid economic growth in Western economies, underpinned by policies based on the ideas of economist John Maynard Keynes, who had argued that governments should play a central role in managing the economy so as to avoid prolonged recessions and keep unemployment low. Welfare states were consolidated in many Western countries, ensuring comprehensive social security and universal health insurance or provision. This 'golden age' for Western economies thus combined trade liberalization and high levels of economic integration with a central role for the state in managing the economy and ensuring the welfare of its citizens.

By the 1970s, however, many Western economies began to experience 'stagflation': a combination of high unemployment (or stagnation) and price increases (inflation). This provided the opportunity for 'neo-liberal' economists to argue that Keynesian policies were the cause of the problem and should be abandoned. The enthusiastic adoption of neo-liberal ideas by leaders such as US President Ronald Reagan and UK Prime Minister Margaret Thatcher in the early 1980s heralded a shift away from state intervention, an erosion of welfare states and a renewed project of economic liberalization. Trade negotiations were intensified, foreign direct investment (FDI) encouraged and financial deregulation policies implemented. These processes were reinforced during the 1980s and 1990s by the collapse of the Soviet Union and the more deliberate integration of China into the world economy. We can see, therefore, that while the integration of national economies was in train in the nineteenth century, and was greatly intensified during the post-Second World War period, contemporary forms of globalization date from the 1980s.

However, the global financial crisis of 2007–2009 dealt a severe blow to the world economy, causing the largest contraction of economic activity since the Great Depression. While in the immediate aftermath of the financial crisis governments implemented coordinated economic stimulus measures, along Keynesian lines, their attention quickly shifted to the resulting growth in government debt. Many governments began to implement 'austerity' policies with the aim of reducing debt.

However, this often led to drastic cuts in public services and welfare provision and had negative effects on economic growth (Farnsworth and Irving 2015). These austerity policies, together with stagnating levels of income for many workers in high-income countries (HICs) and the perception, in the US in particular, that manufacturing jobs had been lost to China and other rapidly developing middle-income countries, led to a growing nationalist backlash against neo-liberal globalization (Rodrik 2018). A referendum in the UK in 2016 saw a small majority vote to leave the EU, while in the US Donald Trump was elected president and quickly set in train a 'trade war' with China that caused massive disruption to global trade. The coronavirus pandemic that began in early 2020 further undermined economic growth as governments' attempts to contain the virus greatly restricted economic activity. These events introduced an element of uncertainty into the global economy and its governance. While economic globalization was not reversed, it was significantly disrupted, and neo-liberal forms of globalization are no longer taken for granted.

Three aspects of economic globalization

Today, economic globalization, and the associated integration between national economies, can be understood in relation to its three main components: trade, FDI and financial globalization.

Trade

Global trade involves the exchange of goods and services between people or entities that reside in different countries. Trade is easiest to understand in relation to goods, although as will be discussed below, services are also traded across borders. Trade occurs where goods produced in one country are shipped to another and sold to consumers residing there. Contemporary patterns of trade result from processes of liberalization, especially in the post-Second World War period, designed to remove barriers to trade (O'Brien and Williams 2020). Trade liberalization can be thought of as the opposite of trade 'protectionism', in which governments erect barriers to trade in an attempt to protect domestic industry and employment from foreign competition. The main barriers to goods trade are tariffs (duties or taxes levied on a good being imported into a country) and quotas (limitations on the quantity or monetary value of a good being imported into a country). Local content requirements, where a government may stipulate that companies must use a minimum percentage of domestically produced components in a product sold within the country, may also be regarded as barriers to goods traded. Substantial liberalization of goods trade took place during the post- Second World War period as a result of the reduction or removal of quotas and the reduction of tariffs, resulting in an increase in the total volume of goods traded. This was facilitated initially via the GATT and, after its creation in 1995, the World Trade Organization (WTO).

Services may also be traded (including health services). Since consumers must often be present in the same place as producers (or 'suppliers') when services are traded, services trade takes different forms to that of goods trade. In its General Agreement on Trade in Services (GATS), the WTO identifies four 'modes of supply' for services trade: (1) cross-border supply, where the supplier and the consumer remain in different countries as in the case of a service provided over the internet; (2) consumption abroad, where the consumer travels to the place where the service is provided; (3) commercial presence, where a supplier from one country establishes or invests in a service outlet within another country (see FDI below); and (4) movement of natural persons, where a professional temporarily moves to another country to provide a service.

Increasingly, as previous trade agreements have been successful in reducing tariffs and quotas, trade negotiations have shifted to include more complex, and often highly controversial, issues that are concerned not with trade in a narrow sense but rather with how governments regulate the goods sold and services provided in their territories. These regulations may be seen as constituting indirect or 'non-tariff' barriers to trade where they have the effect of excluding foreign goods or services that do not (or cannot) meet these standards. Consequently, modern trade agreements have come to include 'behind-the-border' provisions on regulatory cooperation which, along with dispute settlement procedures, many see as reducing governments' 'policy space' to protect the health and well-being of their populations (see Chapter 13).

Foreign direct investment (FDI)

FDI takes place when a person or an entity invests in producing a good or providing a service in a country other than their 'home' country. FDI grew at an even faster rate than trade from the 1980s (Mallampally and Sauvant 1999), reaching annual flows of between $1.5 and $2 trillion during the 2010s (UNCTAD 2021: 2). Most FDI is undertaken by transnational corporations (TNCs), which often have complex global supply chains. TNCs can be extremely large, employing hundreds of thousands of people, with annual turnovers and profits of billions of dollars (Dicken 2014). Processes of merger and acquisition in globalized markets have led many sectors to be dominated by a small number of very large firms. For example, the global tobacco industry is dominated by four large transnational tobacco companies (TTCs), which between them control over 50 per cent of the world market (by volume) outside of China (Hawkins et al. 2018). Acquisition of domestic tobacco companies has been a key strategy of these four TTCs when expanding into new countries (Lee et al. 2013). Trade and FDI are closely related, since both are dominated by TNCs, with approximately 70 per cent of world trade being related to TNCs and about one-third being intra-firm (Lanz and Miroudot 2011). Intra-firm trade takes place where a subsidiary of a TNC trades with another subsidiary of the same TNC.

Financial globalization

The globalization of finance involves the globalization of the banking system (which deals with savings, credit and debt) and an increase in the ease with which currencies and financial assets may be traded across national borders.

Since most countries have their own currencies, for trade to take place one currency must be exchanged for another. The exchange rate, or value at which one currency exchanges with another, can be set in a number of ways. In a fixed exchange rate system, a country's government or central bank attempts to ensure that its currency maintains a specific exchange rate with some other currency or with gold, or at least to limit variations in the exchange rate around a central value so that the exchange rate stays within a narrow band. Since the 1970s, most countries within the global economy have moved to a system of 'floating' exchange rates, meaning that the price of one currency when exchanged with another is determined by supply and demand within financial markets, with only limited intervention by governments to influence exchange rates (Rodrik 2012). The European Union (EU) is unusual in facilitating the adoption of a single currency, the euro, by many different countries in an attempt to overcome the financial instability that can accompany floating exchange rates.

The shift to a predominantly floating exchange rate system globally was accompanied by extensive deregulation of the banking system in many countries, most notably the USA and the UK. Among reforms to the banking system in these countries was the removal of the previously strict separation between retail banking and investment banking, which had been introduced after the Great Depression to protect 'high street' banking for households from the risks of speculative investment (see below). Such reforms increased the complexity of financial markets while facilitating consolidation in the banking industry, so that financial markets became characterized by a number of large global banks.

One aspect of financial globalization, portfolio investment, can be distinguished from FDI in that it is concerned with the purchase of stocks, bonds or other financial assets by financial institutions such as banks on their own behalf or for wealthy clients. Unlike FDI, portfolio investment is not concerned with the direct management of a long-term investment in order to produce a good or provide a service, but rather with an intention to realize a profit from the ownership of a financial asset. Portfolio investment may be of a short-term nature and may be speculative. After the 1970s, a number of influential economists advocated for the abandonment of 'capital controls' that had limited the movement of money across borders and thus restricted the short-term purchase of such assets. As a result of this, 'hot money' – speculative, short-term investments designed to profit from interest rate differences or expected exchange rate movements – became widespread.

From the 1980s onwards, the changes described above combined to create a highly globalized financial system. Information and communication technologies that facilitated the buying and selling of financial assets from anywhere in the world led to a massive increase in the magnitude and speed of financial transactions. While some economists thought that this would lead to a more efficient allocation of resources within the global economy, it produced a much more volatile financial system than that which had existed previously. Financial crises became more common, sweeping through East Asia and Russia in the 1990s and culminating in the global financial crisis of 2007–2009 (Stiglitz 2017).

Global economic governance

A number of intergovernmental organizations (IGOs) play a key role in global economic governance. Three such organizations between them provide the main governance architecture for the world economy: the IMF, the World Bank and the WTO.

The International Monetary Fund (IMF)

The IMF and the World Bank were created at the Bretton Woods conference of 1944. The IMF played the major role in supporting the Bretton Woods monetary system referred to above. Where a country found itself in economic difficulty and incapable of servicing its external debts, it would be able to turn to the IMF for short-term lending and policy advice. The Bretton Woods monetary system was flexible enough to allow for countries to devalue (or revalue) their currencies against the dollar where they were incapable of staying within the agreed exchange rate bands, so long as they did so in an orderly way with the support of the IMF. In order to receive IMF loans a country's government would have to follow the IMF's policy advice in restructuring its economy in a fashion that was deemed to be necessary to allow it to maintain its integration into the world economy and reinsert itself into the monetary system in an orderly way. This is the origin of the lending 'conditionality', which has been one of the most controversial aspects of its work.

With the collapse of the Bretton Woods monetary system in the 1970s, and the shift to floating exchange rates, the IMF retained its central role as lender-of-last-resort to governments. A key period occurred in the 1980s, when a number of Latin American and other countries experienced a debt crisis, with governments unable to service their loans. The IMF, working in parallel with the World Bank, required governments to adopt 'structural adjustment' programmes involving the cutting of public spending, privatization of national assets and liberalization of their economies, in order to stabilize their budgets and the economy more broadly (Anderssen 2020). Such programmes reflected the so-called 'Washington consensus', a set of pro-market ideas promoted by the IMF, the World Bank and the US government, all of which are based in Washington, DC.

Both the macroeconomic effectiveness of such policies and their social effects have been vigorously debated, with some arguing that they failed to protect the poorest citizens of low- and middle-income countries (LMICs) or to generate fair outcomes (Held 2009). The criticisms such policies attracted caused a partial rethink of the types of conditions attached to IMF and World Bank loans (Mosley 2009). However, policy conditionality remains at the heart of the IMF's processes, which attained a new importance in the governance of the global economy following the global financial crisis of 2007–2009. Countries such as Greece that had to seek IMF assistance (alongside that provided by the European Commission and European Central Bank) were required to implement tough 'austerity' policies, with widespread social impacts (Papadopoulos and Roumpakis 2018).

The World Bank

The IMF's 'sister' organization, the World Bank, is actually a group of five distinct organizations. The largest of these, the International Bank for Reconstruction and Development (IBRD) was set up at Bretton Woods with the intention that it would be the means of disbursing American aid for post-war reconstruction in Europe. With the advent of the Marshall Plan, which channelled American aid directly to war-torn European countries, and the post-war process of decolonization in the Global South, the IBRD reoriented its activities towards supporting the economic development of LMICs. Together with another of the organizations within the World Bank group, the International Development Association (IDA), the IBRD provides low-cost loans to LMICs for development purposes.

Stung by the criticisms of structural adjustment processes in the 1980s, and in particular the impact upon the poorest citizens of LMICs, the World Bank has since reoriented itself to also become a 'knowledge bank'. It now puts the reduction and abolition of extreme poverty globally at the centre of its mission, situating itself as the foremost repository of data and expertise on global poverty. Like the IMF, it continues to attach conditions to its loans, but these now include a requirement that the poorest citizens should be protected during processes of economic restructuring. Both the Bank's focus on the very poorest (rather than on more comprehensive social protection policies) and its methods of measuring extreme poverty have been subject to criticism (Holden 2022). Nevertheless, it does provide important data on trends in extreme poverty that are central to measuring the progress of the Sustainable Development Goals (SDGs), which we will discuss in the final section of this chapter.

The World Trade Organization (WTO)

Following its creation in 1995, the WTO assumed responsibility for the GATT and a range of new trade agreements, including the GATS, that were agreed during the Uruguay round of trade negotiations (1986–1993). The WTO, like the GATT system before it, works to reduce trade barriers through a series of negotiating rounds between its member states, with the intention of creating a rules-based system within which trade can take place. While the WTO remains central to processes of trade liberalization at the global level, there is also a large range of regional and bilateral trade agreements and organizations that operate outside of the auspices of the WTO. The functioning and health effects of WTO and other trade agreements are discussed further in Chapter 13.

✎ Activity 2.3

Using the websites of the World Bank and the IMF, find out how each one is organized. How are member states represented within each organization? Does voting take place in any of the organization's bodies? If so, on what basis? Which member states would you say have most influence within the organization?

Feedback

The IMF and the World Bank are organized in a very similar way, with member-state voting rights on important issues varying by quotas (for the IMF) or shares (in the five component parts of the World Bank Group). This means that HICs, particularly the USA, have much more influence than low-income countries. However, IGOs can be organized in a wide variety of ways; the WTO, for example, is organized very differently to the IMF and the World Bank.

Poverty, inequality and economic development

In addition to the roles that IGOs such as those discussed above play in global governance, the United Nations (UN) system oversees a set of global goals that governments and IGOs aim to work towards. These are the SDGs, which superseded the Millennium Development Goals (MDGs) in 2015. There are 17 SDGs, each of which has its own targets and indicators. Foremost is Goal 1, which commits governments and UN organizations to 'end poverty in all its forms everywhere'. Despite the headline commitment to end poverty 'in all its forms', the priority is Goal 1, Target 1.1, which is aimed at the eradication of *extreme* poverty. Progress towards this target is measured by the World Bank's primary measure of global poverty, the 'international poverty line', which is currently set at $1.90 a day. The 'abolition' of extreme poverty is operationalized as aiming at its reduction by this measure to 3 per cent or less of the world's population. Additionally, SDG Goal 10 aims to 'reduce inequality within and among countries', with Target 10.1 aiming to 'progressively achieve and sustain income growth of the bottom 40 per cent of the population at a rate higher than the national average'.

Using the international poverty line, World Bank data show that there has been substantial progress towards Target 1.1, with a consistent reduction in extreme poverty since 1990 (see, for example, World Bank 2018). World Bank analysts tend to argue that this positive trend indicates the success of economic liberalization policies that have increased the openness of a number of LMIC economies to the global economy during the relevant period and thereby stimulated economic growth. However, a closer look at the data suggests a more nuanced picture. The overall downward trend in extreme poverty is disproportionately influenced by rapid economic growth in China, which did indeed experience a process of sustained opening of its economy from the 1990s onwards. Yet many countries have not experienced such spectacular growth as a result of liberalization policies, prompting some economists to argue that a 'one size fits all' approach to economic policy is inappropriate (Rodrik 2007).

Furthermore, where economic growth and the reduction of extreme poverty have occurred, they have often been accompanied by a growth in inequality, as the gains of growth are disproportionately captured by those at the top of the income distribution (Holden 2022).

Further reduction of poverty and an attempt to tackle growing inequality are, therefore, dependent on government social policies to provide adequate social protection systems and to ensure the fairer distribution of the proceeds of economic growth. The World Bank (2018) itself had already noted prior to the Covid-19 pandemic that, assuming a continuation of trend rates of economic growth, such growth would be insufficient to achieve the global abolition of extreme poverty by the proposed deadline unless accompanied by government policies to tackle inequality. Moreover, the Covid-19 pandemic has had a profound negative impact on growth rates in most countries and, therefore, on rates of poverty reduction. The policies that governments adopt in the wake of the pandemic will thus be crucial in determining future trends in poverty and inequality.

✏ Activity 2.4

Go to the pages on the World Bank's website that focus on global poverty (https://globalization.worldbank.org/en/understanding-poverty). Look for different estimates of global poverty using different global poverty lines, including the World Bank's extreme poverty measure, the international poverty line. How do rates of poverty differ between countries and world regions? How do poverty rates change depending on which poverty measure is used? Which countries or regions account for the greatest and smallest reductions in poverty?

Feedback

Reduction in extreme poverty between 1990 and 2020 was greatest in the East Asian region, mainly due to robust economic growth in China, and lowest in Sub-Saharan Africa, for a variety of reasons, including the incidence of conflict in many countries. The most up-to-date estimates show how the Covid-19 pandemic may affect long-term trends in different countries and regions.

Summary

National economies became increasingly integrated with each other during the nineteenth century. This integration was disrupted by the two world wars and the Great Depression, but increased in pace after the Second World War. Economic globalization increased further from the 1980s, facilitated by policies of trade, investment and financial liberalization. Economic liberalization policies can promote economic growth and thereby reduce poverty in some cases, but such policies need to be tailored to the specific needs of each country. Governments' social policies are crucial in shaping how the proceeds of economic growth are distributed among their populations and how economic processes influence health outcomes. Global economic governance is overseen by a variety of IGOs, the most important of which are the IMF, the World Bank and the WTO. The roles of IGOs in global health are discussed in Chapter 10, while the implications of WTO and other trade agreements for public health are explored further in Chapter 13.

References

Andersson, E. (2020) *Reconstructing the Global Political Economy: An Analytical Guide*. Bristol: Bristol University Press.

Dicken, P. (2014) *Global Shift: Mapping the Changing Contours of the World Economy*, 7th edn, London: Sage.

Farnsworth, K. and Irving, Z. (eds) (2015) *Social Policy in Times of Austerity: Global Economic Crisis and the New Politics of Welfare*. Bristol: Policy Press.

Galbraith, J.K. (2009) *The Great Crash 1929*. London: Penguin.

Hawkins, B., Holden, C., Eckhardt, J. et al. (2018) Reassessing policy paradigms: a comparison of the global tobacco and alcohol industries, *Global Public Health*, 13(1): 1–19.

Held, D. (2009) At the global crossroads (Part A): the end of the Washington Consensus?, in N. Yeates and C. Holden (eds) *The Global Social Policy Reader*. Bristol: Policy Press.

Hirst, P., Thompson, G. and Bromley, S. (2009) *Globalization in Question*, 3rd edn, Cambridge: Polity Press.

Holden, C. (2022) Global poverty and inequality, in N. Yeates and C. Holden (eds) *Understanding Global Social Policy*. Bristol: Policy Press.

Lanz, R. and Miroudot, S. (2011) *Intra-firm Trade: Patterns, Determinants and Policy Implications, OECD Trade Policy Papers*, No. 114. Paris: OECD Publishing.

Lee, S., Holden, C. and Lee, K. (2013) Are transnational tobacco companies' market access strategies linked to economic development models? A case study of South Korea, *Global Public Health*, 8(4): 435–448.

Mallampally, P. and Sauvant, K.P. (1999) Foreign direct investment in developing countries, *Finance & Development*, 36(1): 34–37.

Marx, K. and Engels, F. (2018 [1848]) *The Communist Manifesto*. London: Penguin.

Mosley, P. (2009) Attacking poverty and the 'Post-Washington Consensus', in N. Yeates and C. Holden (eds) *The Global Social Policy Reader*. Bristol: Policy Press.

O'Brien, R. and Williams, M. (2020) *Global Political Economy: Evolution and Dynamics*, 6th edn. London: Red Globe Press.

Papadopoulos, T. and Roumpakis, A. (2018) Rattling Europe's ordoliberal 'iron cage': the contestation of austerity in Southern Europe, *Critical Social Policy*, 38(3): 505–526.

Rodrik, D. (2007) *One Economics, Many Recipes: Globalization, Institutions and Economic Growth*. Princeton, NJ: Princeton University Press.

Rodrik, D. (2012) *The Globalization Paradox: Why Global Markets, States and Democracy Can't Coexist*. Oxford: Oxford University Press.

Rodrik, D. (2018) Populism and the economics of globalization, *Journal of International Business Policy*, 1(1–2): 12–33.

Stiglitz, J. (2017) *Globalization and its Discontents Revisited: Anti-Globalization in the Era of Trump*. London: Penguin.

UNCTAD (2021) *World Investment Report 2021*. New York: United Nations Conference on Trade and Investment.

World Bank (2018) *Piecing Together the Poverty Puzzle*. Washington, DC: World Bank.

Globalization, social change and health

3

Donald Brown and Carolyn Stephens

Overview

Globalization is a process that influences all areas of human life. Chapter 2 focused on economic changes, but globalization has a much wider impact on society, reshaping our lives and our relationships with each other. This chapter explores how globalization is changing aspects of our social lives, linked to demographic, technological and economic changes, with significant implications for health. Particular attention is paid to the interconnections between globalization and urbanization, and the consequences not only for the social determinants of health but also for the norms and values that shape the way people from different socio-economic backgrounds and geographic locations see, experience and participate in the world.

Learning objectives

After working through this chapter, you will be able to:

- Identify social changes linked to globalization and explore key concepts to help understand these changes.
- Understand the varying impacts these social changes may have on the social determinants of health.

Key terms

Global village: The idea that globalization is compressing space and time, creating a shared experience across nation states and cultural boundaries.

Social determinants of health: The idea that social conditions can determine the ways in which people grow, work and live, and that these conditions influence health both directly and indirectly.

Cognitive impacts of globalization: The idea that globalization is creating shifts in the ways in which we think about each other and in how our ideas, aspirations and consumption patterns are formed.

Global citizen: The idea that there are people who identify with shared global notions of citizenship rather than, or in addition to, allegiance to any cultural, religious, linguistic or national identity.

Urban social change: The idea that globalization combines with other processes of socio-demographic change to re-shape the social structures of urban populations.

Conceptualizing social change and health in the context of globalization

As other chapters in this textbook describe, globalization is often discussed in terms of global trade (Chapter 13), or macro-economic (Chapter 2), environmental (Chapter 7), and governance (Chapter 4) changes. It is also fundamentally about our social lives and connections globally, and our shared values and aspirations – or not. Presciently, the sociologist Anthony Giddens noted in a 1999 Reith lecture for the British national broadcasting company: 'It is wrong to think of globalization as just concerning the big systems, like the world financial order. Globalization isn't only about what is "out there", remote and far away from the individual. It is an "in here" phenomenon too, influencing intimate and personal aspects of our lives' (Giddens 1999; Giddens 2002).

A powerful concept linking social change to globalization is that of a 'global village' and perhaps, as evocatively, the idea of 'global citizens'. Both of these notions encapsulate the idea that people are living beyond boundaries – and these could be national, cultural, linguistic, religious, ethnic or any other boundaries we construct or perceive to be between each other. Global citizens, living in this global village, are presumed to share values and beliefs, a common global citizenship and shared aspirations. This is a relatively attractive idea – it is mirrored in many of our global institutions (such as the United Nations) and many of our global treaties and declarations (such as the UN Declaration on Human Rights). However, even as we look at the positive aspects of these ideas, we need to explore the nature of the social changes occurring in where we live, how we work and how we interact, and the different impacts that globalization is having on different people across the world. These include the process of urbanization, with changes in living conditions and livelihoods, and also changes in our values, norms and our social relationships. They also include social counter-trends – which seem to challenge the idea of global villages, or global citizenship, which is explored in Chapter 1 and Chapter 14.

Health is shaped by 'the conditions in which people are born, grow, live, work and age' (WHO 2008); we call these conditions the social determinants of health. These social conditions mediate the overall political and economic structures of our societies: for example, political and economic integration linked with globalization is experienced according to the specific conditions of where we live, where we work and who we are surrounded by.

WHO sees these social determinants of health as the non-medical factors that influence health outcomes (WHO 2021). These include:

- Income and social protection
- Education
- Unemployment and job insecurity
- Working life conditions
- Food insecurity
- Housing, basic amenities and the environment
- Early childhood development
- Social inclusion and non-discrimination
- Structural conflict
- Access to affordable health services of decent quality

The interplay of these factors is key and changes greatly in different contexts. This makes the assessment of the health impacts of social determinants very difficult. The links between these changes and the process of globalization are also highly complex. However, one thing is clear: the levels of social and economic inequalities within societies link closely to the pattern of social determinants of health (WHO 2021). In recognition of this, several governments, and academics globally, have now started to explore and adapt the WHO social determinants framework to their own contexts (see, e.g. Omotoso and Koch 2018).

It is important also to put any discussion of social change and social determinants of health in historical context. Societies all over the world have evolved from a long history of change including cultural, religious and territorial shifts over millennia – some peaceful transitions and some violent impositions of one culture over another. A clear and relatively recent manifestation of the imposition of one set of cultures over many others is the (largely) European colonization of vast territories of Africa, Asia and Latin America (UN 2021). This has had lasting and ongoing repercussions for the peoples of colonized countries, including social repercussions in terms of language, culture and, in many settings, religion, values and norms. In Chapter 10 we will discuss current bilateral and multilateral actors, but it is important to note that we are now in the fourth international decade (2021–2030) for the eradication of colonialism, a process overseen by a special committee of the United Nations. Since the birth of the United Nations, more than 80 former colonies comprising some 750 million people have gained independence. At present, however, there are still 17 Non-Self-Governing Territories (NSGTs), defined as territories whose people have not yet attained a full measure of self-government. These territories are home to nearly 2 million people. Thus, the UN committee notes that 'the process of decolonization is not complete' (UN 2021). We will discuss the links of colonialism with globalization in other chapters, but here we are concerned with the ongoing legacy of colonialism in social values and norms and the ways in which colonial relations can interact with global changes affecting people's lives and opportunities.

There are also important socio-demographic differences between societies – for example, the degree of urbanization, of conflict or inequality. Particular groups in a society, for example indigenous peoples in some contexts, might have a very different set of social determinants to their health and might also understand these determinants in a different way. For example, cultural and social identity for many indigenous peoples is linked to their natural world, and access to, and the health of, traditional lands are considered important determinants of health (Stephens 2020). These differences between contexts mean that it is inevitable that social changes linked to globalization are highly complex and differ greatly in different settings. As Chapter 2 explains, globalization is creating enormous differences in material wealth and opportunity, which are linked to increases in health inequities in almost all countries. The implications of this may also play out in very different ways in different settings.

✎ Activity 3.1 Globalization – shifting social determinants

The WHO Commission on Social Determinants of Health showed how important non-medical factors are for human health. Explore the list on page 33. Taking TWO of the non-medical factors, explore how you think these affect your health or those of your community.

Feedback

When you start to think about your health and the non-medical factors described by WHO, you will see how difficult it is to link social circumstances directly to health outcomes. Some aspects of our lives are easier to relate to our health. For example, living conditions, particularly if they are precarious, can be a major determinant of poor health outcomes. But when you think about why someone is in precarious living conditions, you need to consider the complex social history and chain of structural inequalities underlying these conditions – perhaps you think about educational opportunities, which might be limited or non-existent; in turn, these might lead to insecure, low paid work – which then might only allow people to live in cheaper, often precarious living conditions. Working life conditions may be hazardous and directly expose people to health risks. But then if you explore the social context that leads people to need to take hazardous jobs, you start to unpack the social determinants of their working lives and health risks. Some working life conditions may be also unhealthy directly because they are stressful and insecure, and cause anxiety and consequent health impacts. Overall, relating poor health outcomes to social aspects of your society, your employment status, or history is highly complex. Social changes linked to globalization are long-term contextual and historical processes. This leads to a fundamental challenge with trying to track the causal path from social circumstances to health outcomes. This becomes even more challenging when you try to link global processes to social changes and then to health. Challenging as it is, trying to trace these links is key to understanding the health impacts of globalization.

Key dimensions and concepts of social change

In the following sections, we start with shifting socio-spatial conditions and shifting livelihoods, and then look at shifts in ways of interacting and communicating and shifts in norms and values. For each of these areas we will discuss the social processes affected by globalization and their impact on health.

Shifting socio-spatial conditions

People have always moved within and across borders in response to various push factors (such as wars, disasters and famine) and pull factors (such as employment opportunities and better lifestyles). While migration is not a new phenomenon, globalization has increased population movement through advancements in technology and transportation alongside the quest for better jobs and services, including healthcare (IOM 2020). As economic activities and new technologies have spread across the globe, people have increasingly moved to cities. So, in many senses globalization has accelerated urbanization, increasing the share of people in urban living environments and transforming how people live, work and interact socially (WHO and UN-Habitat 2016).

In 2018, 55 per cent of the world population lived in urban areas and this proportion is projected to rise to 70 per cent by 2050 (UNDESA 2019). This demographic shift is global in scale but geographically uneven. Europe and North America alongside Latin America and the Caribbean are now predominately urban, with more than 75 per cent of their populations living in towns and cities (UNDESA 2019). Africa and Asia are the most rapidly urbanizing continents and are doing so under different global economic conditions. The advanced economies have lost much of their manufacturing industry and have been forced to undergo economic restructuring toward service industries, as observed in the 'rust-belt cities' of the mid-West United States. The continent that currently benefits most from globalized urban development is Asia (Trujillo and Parilla 2016). Meanwhile, Africa has been largely bypassed by the global economic system, though a small number of large metropolitan centres (notably Cairo, Dakar, Johannesburg, Nairobi and Lagos) have recently emerged as regional economic hubs (Parnell and Simon 2014).

The increasing share of people in urban living environments does not imply a shift away from rural areas. Urbanization and globalization can intensify rural-urban flows and interactions involving people, income (via remittances), trade, information, technology, ecosystem services and environmental problems. For example: high-density rural areas called 'desakotas' (from the Indonesian words *desa* 'village' and *kota* 'city') have emerged due to the expansion and influence of metropolitan economies, as observed in East and Southeast Asia; urban growth has increased dependence on ecological services from rural hinterlands and more distant 'elsewheres'; and persistent urban economic instability in low-income regions (notably Southeast Asia and sub-Saharan Africa) has led to circular migration trends (rural–urban–rural) as a livelihood diversification strategy (UN-Habitat 2008).

The 40 largest mega-city regions generate two-thirds of global economic output, but accommodate just 18 per cent of the world's population (Trujillo and Parilla 2016). Many more urban dwellers live in small and intermediate urban centres (with less than 500,000 inhabitants), which account for a large and generally growing share of the world's urban growth – a trend that is projected to continue (urban population statistics are regularly updated by the United Nations, see UNDESA 2019). These smaller centres play key roles in regional development through connecting rural localities with domestic and global markets for agricultural products and through providing non-farm employment opportunities. They are important social hubs also, bringing together rural peoples from the surrounding hinterlands. But they tend to lack strong local governments and be politically and economically weak, with their populations often in unhealthy living environments (UN-Habitat 2020a).

Furthermore, refugees and internally displaced persons (IDPs) increasingly settle in cities rather than traditional camp settings due to the availability of urban livelihood opportunities and services – another trend that is projected to continue (UNHCR 2018). In these urban settlements, the displaced often face a triple-burden of infectious disease (e.g. tuberculosis, hepatitis), chronic disease (e.g. diabetes, respiratory problems) and mental health conditions (e.g. depression, post-traumatic stress disorder) (Abbas et al. 2018). As a result, protracted displacement has created major challenges for local authorities, host communities and humanitarian agencies struggling to adjust to the added pressures, including on social and health services.

Linked to increased population movement, urban areas often contain a very diverse mix of people with multiple intersecting identities (e.g. gender, ethnicity/race, religion, nationality) and statuses (e.g. formal/informal labourer, migrant/non-migrant, citizen/non-citizen) (UN-Habitat 2020b: 169–173). Global change has contributed to this diversity, which is often seen as a manifestation of more inclusive societies (the 'global village'). However, the urban experience depends very much on the socio-economic conditions of the urban residents. Many newcomers are from excluded social groups, face marginalization and discrimination in the labour market and have limited access to resources, notably affordable housing and services. In China, for example, rural to urban migrants have long faced barriers to accessing health and other social services in urban destinations, and the migration process may expose them to greater health risks and inequities (Zheng et al. 2020). This phenomenon is also observed among recent newcomers in European and North American cities, such as Toronto in Canada (Ahmadi 2018).

Because globalization often contributes to socio-spatial exclusion in cities, it has been associated with increasing urban poverty and inequality. This is linked to the concurrent growth of informal settlements and 'slums' with health and life-threatening conditions, which have become the norm in much of the Global South (Ezeh et al. 2017). But the socio-economic impacts of globalized urbanization are not only negative; they can also be positive owing to the concentration of resources, livelihood opportunities, markets and services (including healthcare) in urban areas. The positive aspects of urban living contribute to the so-called 'urban advantage', whereby urban dwellers generally enjoy better health than their rural counterparts (WHO and UN-Habitat 2016). In reality, however, the depth of urban inequality means that low-income groups often suffer from an 'urban penalty' (WHO and UN-Habitat 2010).

✐ Activity 3.2

Consider the advantages that urban environments (in terms of labour markets, services, social networks, etc.) confer on the health of urban dwellers. Do the urban poor enjoy these advantages to the same degree? If not, what are the key barriers that prevent different peoples living in urban poverty from living healthy lives?

Feedback

In urban areas, the costs of accessing non-food essentials (notably housing and services, such as water) are monetized. To pay for these costs, urban dwellers must earn an income. Those with low incomes will struggle to make ends meet, especially where a large share of income is spent on housing. Without viable alternatives, the urban poor often live in settlements (typically informal) with very poor housing and living conditions. Where these settlements are viewed by officials as 'illegal', the urban poor may be denied secure land tenure (in the form of formal land titles), basic services (including water and sanitation), the rule of law and access to decision-making. So rather than enjoying an 'urban advantage', the urban poor often suffer from an 'urban penalty' associated with unsanitary, insecure and unsafe living conditions – conditions especially pronounced in the low- and middle-income countries.

The urban poor should not be treated as a homogeneous group. Some people are more vulnerable to poverty-related disease based on their socio-economic status and geographic location. So any analysis of the links between urban poverty and health must take a disaggregated approach, whereby health is seen as socio-spatially differentiated.

The impacts of globalization are not just confined to urban areas. Globalization is a process that involves the stretching and strengthening of social, economic and cultural relations across space, integrating even the most distant places in global and regional networks (Woods 2017). The impacts of this process can be positive, as where migrants transfer large amounts of income, wealth, information and ideas to their rural localities of origin. The impacts can be negative also, as where the extension of global supply chains into food and agriculture has weakened the social relations between local communities and farmers. So, globalization and urbanization should not be conflated, even though they have strong inter-connections.

Shifting livelihoods

Globalization has, arguably, created job opportunities, more financial security and raised incomes for the newly urbanized billions, although the benefits have not been equally distributed (Schrecker 2009). In high-income countries, economic restructuring has led to the creation of knowledge-intensive services (particularly in the finance, information and technology sectors) and a highly skilled labour force based in cities. But as global capital and labour have become increasingly footloose, the links between occupational stratification and socio-spatial inequalities have intensified (Sassen 2001). In Toronto, for example, immigrants have long provided a pool of inexpensive labour forced to accept low-paying and low-skill jobs in the service sector, such as housekeeping, catering, transport and care work (Joy and Vogel 2015). Meanwhile, the concentration of professional services and head offices in central areas has created a growing number of knowledge workers who have gentrified the inner-city core, displacing recent newcomers and ethnic minority groups into outlying areas (Joy and Vogel 2015).

The relocation of manufacturing to low- and middle-income countries is another important trend associated with globalization, which has created low-wage jobs (often informal) with minimal protection (Schrecker 2009). Informal employment accounts for more than 50 per cent of non-agricultural employment (typically urban) in most of the world's low- to middle-income countries and substantially more in those regions that are urbanizing: upwards of 80 per cent in parts of sub-Saharan Africa and South Asia (data on the share of informal employment by region are regularly updated by the ILO – for example, ILO 2021). Globalization has contributed to the growth of the informal economy, particularly where production has been outsourced to informal enterprises through global supply chains (as in the case of the fashion garment industry). Working conditions are particularly poor in the informal sector due generally to exposure to chemical pollutants and accidental injuries, long hours, low pay and the absence of health and safety standards (WHO and UN-Habitat 2010).

Increased competition for mobile capital and labour between countries and individual urban centres has led to the deregulation of the business environment (Harvey 1989). The 'race to the bottom' describes the resulting impacts on low wages, environmental degradation and other externalities. The evidence indicates that the socio-economic benefits of globalization are rapidly being offset by the negative impacts of poorly planned urbanization and rising urban poverty, especially among women (UN-Habitat 2004, 2013).

✎ Activity 3.3

Consider the health risks and opportunities that might be faced by a young woman moving to an urban area in search of work. How would these differ from those faced by men?

Feedback

Urban women generally enjoy more socio-economic advantages than their rural counterparts. Such advantages include better access to healthcare (including reproductive services), education, livelihoods and greater autonomy from wage earning. While these advantages pose clear health benefits, not all urban women enjoy them to the same degree. Gender inequalities prevent women from participating in the labour market, moving freely outside the home and wider city, and gaining representation in urban governance. Consequent physical and mental health risks range from unsafe working conditions to sexual violence, fear and insecurity, and a double burden of productive and domestic work. For slum-dwelling women, these risks are amplified by poor housing and living conditions, such as where dirty fuels are used for cooking in homes lacking ventilation. Or where unreliable water supplies force women to use alternative sources in distant locations, often using precarious footpaths.

Shifting relationships and communication

The idea of a global village was first conceived to describe a global community of people living in different places across the world – the so-called network society (Castells 2009). Central to this concept is one of the key elements of globalization – technological change – and, in this case, information technology, linked to massive changes in the social lives of billions of people around the world. The changes in the ways in which we communicate started in the nineteenth century with the advent of the telegraph and have accelerated significantly in the late twentieth and early twenty-first centuries – with the evolution and wide diffusion of communication technologies and internet access – even for remote communities and individuals (Stephens 2020).

Fundamentally, information technology, as all technologies, could be thought of as socially 'neutral' – although, in practice, technologies often embody values and even ideologies in their design and material properties. Perhaps the key social aspect of information technologies, and their impacts on the social determinants of health, derives from their use. Information technology and communication can thus be seen as facilitating the benefits of the global society; these range from the more obvious benefits such as access to knowledge and building and facilitating friendships across physical space, to complex benefits such as promoting transparency and accountability through the dissemination of information regarding public and private actors. Simultaneously, information technology can be used to facilitate elites to further their interests and exacerbate divisions between peoples. Over half the world's population are now estimated to have mobile phones, internet connections and be social media users (Wearesocial 2021). Use of these communication tools can include participation in informal 'friendship' networks; online non-governmental lobbying networks; news and information access and consumption of goods and services. Information technologies can also give isolated and socially disenfranchised communities access to the means to communicate their problems – for example, indigenous peoples globally have become very astute in using information technologies to make visible their situation and to share their wisdom with other peoples (Stephens 2020).

Linked to this explosion of communication possibilities is the idea of global citizenship – which is a complex idea given that the term citizen is usually framed as membership of a nation state, with rights conferred by birth or being given due to living/working in that location. It is challenging to think about what a global citizen might look like and how membership of this global citizenry might be linked to global health. Perhaps one interesting example has emerged around UN efforts to tap global consciousness on priority issues including climate change – which has major implications for human health now and in the future. The United Nations is increasingly appealing to the 'global citizen' for opinions and priorities. In 2020, marking the 75th anniversary of the UN, 1.5 million people from all 193 United Nations Member States were asked to give their views on the future and how all actors, including the UN could work together to face global challenges (UN 2021). Also, in 2021, the UN published another global 'poll' which they termed the 'Peoples' Climate Vote' – using the language of voting as if all global citizens were in the position to vote for global issues (UNDP and University of Oxford 2021).

The idea of global citizenship is not without problems – at both conceptual and practical levels. As we have seen in the previous section, the majority of people in the world live and work in really challenging social and economic situations – many of them in the informal sector. In these contexts, connection to the internet, and the time and resources to engage in global debates remain truly available – or perhaps even of interest – to relatively few people. There has been a proliferation of information alongside the increase in use of these information technologies – and with it distrust of some of the sources of this information. Social factors such as language or culture also influence the sources of information that people access or trust. This can affect something as important as trust in fundamental global public health interventions. In 2014, WHO produced an important report on vaccine hesitancy (WHO 2014) and in 2019, for the first time, WHO ranked vaccine hesitancy, linked in part to lack of confidence, as one of 10 global public challenges facing the world (WHO 2019).

The idea of the global citizen assumes that we can all share some important values and aspirations across social, economic, cultural, language, gender and any other difference – the UN is mandated and organized on this premise. But we need to be aware that information technologies can be, and are, used to disseminate and incite violence between peoples on the basis of their socio-cultural characteristics – against refugees for example, or specific minorities in a community. It can also mean that, at an individual level, these technologies can be used for bullying and psychosocial aggression leading to substantial mental health problems for affected individuals. In 2019, UNICEF's 'U-report' highlighted both the risks and the benefits of information technologies: U-report is itself an online information technology that helps young people to report bullying – and more than a third of children in 30 countries reported being victims of online bullying (https://globalization.ureport.in).

✏ **Activity 3.4**

Do you think you live in a global village? In what ways do you feel connected to people globally? Are there peoples in your society or others that you can see as having a different perspective to you on this concept? Can you see any links of this to your health – and how does this differ for other peoples?

Feedback

You may have considered your own life, and very often, as you may be reading this as a post-graduate or graduate student, you may have decided that the idea of the global village is a very familiar and accessible idea to you. You may have identified links to your mental health and well-being. You may have explored the fact that your social life and experiences are relatively privileged compared to some other peoples in your own society or other societies in the world. You may have considered the social position of other peoples in your society and if and why they might perceive the global village differently. You might have reflected also on the perspectives of those who might feel antagonistic to the idea of the global village – and considered why they might feel this way.

Shifting norms and values

In this final section, we discuss trends in communication and relationships that can be associated with globalization. In particular, this section explores whether norms and values are changing. Many see globalization as leading to an integrated global economy. Intrinsic to this is the idea of a 'standardizing' trend, with diverse global cultures becoming more similar, particularly in terms of consumption – including consumption of food, alcohol, dress and even cultural goods such as language and behaviours. The term 'McDonaldization' is one label given to this process – affecting even arts and music (Kabanda 2015).

In many senses, this is the idea of the global citizen from the perspective of consumption. These culturally homogenizing trends – particularly affecting the urban populations discussed earlier – are largely mediated by global corporations that reach global audiences through the same information technologies that we discussed in the previous section. The influence of these trends on health are discussed more fully in later chapters. The factors behind this shift are complex and a major field of economic and anthropological analysis.

These trends impact on lifestyles and behaviours through what can be seen as a methodical attempt to influence what people want and aspire to.

For example, marketing messages globally give meanings to people's lives and may put pressure to fit, or to aspire to fit, a particular idea of the perfect global citizen – from a consumption perspective (Carrier 2021a). For example, this marketing may tell you what will make you look more socially attractive to other people, or how you can fit in with your society, or even aspire to live like members of the elite global society, whose members and lives you can access through information technologies. This is not a new process, but again, it has accelerated and proliferated with information technology. It is also linked to urbanization and the accessibility and 'permeability' of the urban citizen to these messages (Taylor et al. 2020). This process is not necessarily negative or bad for health. Information about products and cultural goods helps us to make informed decisions. Chapter 6 will discuss the impacts of these trends on NCDs. Here the most important concern is about the ways in which these decisions divide people into different groups (largely based on their consumption habits) in ways which may carry moral weight and judgement of worth (Carrier 2021b). What can be termed the 'globalization of aspiration' can be seen to drive a model towards endless upward consumption of products – linked to a social construction of personal worth linked to this. And notably the majority of global citizens have little access to the goods they are being told to aspire to. This has implications for health and for the planet. Notably, in 2020 UNDP modified its ground-breaking Human Development Index (HDI) to add a measure of the impact of a country's population impact on the planet – called the Planetary pressures–adjusted Human Development Index. This comes 30 years after the first HDI was launched to add social aspects of development to broaden our global measurement of human progress (UNDP 2020). We will explore this more in Chapter 7.

Summary

In this chapter, we have explored how globalization is leading to social changes, and so having an effect on the social determinants of health. These determinants will be explored further in later chapters. We have also introduced the ideas of shifting demographic and socio-political conditions, and the ideas of the global village and global citizen. We have described the shifts in norms and values that are taking place and the ways in which we communicate and relate to each other are changing. The ideas and concepts introduced in this chapter can be useful for understanding the underlying social drivers of some of the shifts in health risks that we will explore in the following chapters.

References

Abbas, M., Aloudat, T., Bartolomei, J. et al. (2018) Migrant and refugee populations: a public health and policy perspective on a continuing global crisis, *Antimicrobial Resistance and Infection Control*, 7(113): 1–11.

Ahmadi, D. (2018) Is diversity our strength? An analysis of the facts and fancies of diversity in Toronto, *City, Culture and Society*, 13: 64–72.

Carrier, J.G. (2021a) Consumption and meaning, in J.G. Carrier (ed.) *Economic Anthropology*. Newcastle upon Tyne: Agenda Publishing.

Carrier, J.G. (2021b) Consumption in context, in J.G. Carrier (ed.) *Economic Anthropology*. Newcastle upon Tyne: Agenda Publishing.

Castells, M. (2009) *The Rise of the Network Society*, 2nd edn. Oxford: Wiley Publishers.

Ezeh, A., Oyebode, O., Satterthwaite, D. et al. (2017) The history, geography, and sociology of slums and the health problems of people who live in slums, *The Lancet*, 389(10068): 547–558.

Giddens, A. (1999) Runaway World BBC Reith Lectures episode 1 Globalization, BBC. Available at: https://globalization.bbc.co.uk/programmes/p00gw9s1 (accessed 1 May 2021).

Giddens, A. (2002) *Runaway World: How Globalization is Reshaping Our Lives*. New York: Routledge.

Harvey, D. (1989) From managerialism to entrepreneurialism: the transformation in urban governance in late capitalism, *Geografiska Annaler. Series B, Human Geography*, 71(1): 3–17.

ILO (2021) ILOSTAT: statistics on the informal economy, ILO. Available at: https://ilostat.ilo.org/topics/informality/ (accessed 2 May 2021).

IOM (2020) *World Migration Report 2020*. Grand-Saconnex: United Nations, International Organization for Migration.

Joy, M. and Vogel, R.K. (2015) Toronto's governance crisis: a global city under pressure, *Cities*, 49: 35–52.

Kabanda, P. (2015) *Work as Art: Links between Creative Work and Human Development*. New York: United Nations Development Programme.

Omotoso, K.O. and Koch, S.F. (2018) Assessing changes in social determinants of health inequalities in South Africa: a decomposition analysis, *International Journal for Equity in Health*, 17(181): 1–13.

Parnell, S. and Simon, D. (2014) National urbanisation and urban strategies: necessary but absent policy instruments in Africa, in S. Parnell and E. Pieterse (eds) *Africa's Urban Revolution*. New York: Zed Books.

Sassen, S. (2001) Cities in the global economy, in R. Paddison (ed.) *Handbook of Urban Studies*. New York: Sage Publications.

Schrecker, T. (2009) Labour markets, equity and social determinants of health, in C. Packer and V. Runnels (eds) *Globalization and Health: Pathways, Evidence, Policy*. London: Routledge.

Stephens, C. (2020) The challenges of technology and sustainable development, *Minority and Indigenous Trends 2020*. London: Minority Rights International. Available at: https://minorityrights.org/trends2020/ (accessed 3 May 2021).

Taylor, P.J., O'Brien, G. and O'Keefe, P. (2020) Action: can we stop terminal consumption, in P.J. Taylor, G. O'Brien and P. O'Keefe (eds) *Cities Demanding the Earth: A New Understanding of the Climate Emergency*. Bristol: Bristol University Press.

Trujillo, J. and Parilla, J. (2016) *Redefining Global Cities: The Seven Types of Global Metro Economies*, Metropolitan Policy Program. Washington, DC: The Brookings Institute. Available at: https://globalization.brookings.edu/research/redefining-global-cities/ (accessed 4 May 2021).

UN (2021) *Shaping Our Future Together: Listening to People's Priorities for the Futrue and their Ideas for Action*. New York: United Nations. Available at: https://globalization.un.org/sites/un2.un.org/files/un75_final_report_shapingourfuturetogether.pdf (accessed 18 May 2021).

UNDESA (2019) *United Nations Population Division. World Population Prospects: 2019 Revision*. New York: United Nations Department of Economic and Social Affairs. Available at: https://population.un.org/wpp/ (accessed 27 April 2021).

UNDP (2020) *Human Development Report 2020: The Next Frontier Human Development and the Anthropocene*, United Nations Development Programme Available at: http://hdr.undp.org/sites/default/files/hdr2020.pdf (accessed 18 May 2021).

UNDP and University of Oxford (2021) *People's Climate Vote*. New York and Oxford: United Nations Development Programme and University of Oxford. Available at: https://globalization.undp.org/content/dam/undp/library/km-qap/UNDP-Oxford-Peoples-Climate-Vote-Results.pdf (accessed 17 May 2021).

UN-Habitat (2004) *The State of the World's Cities 2004/2005: Globalization and Urban Culture*. Nairobi: UN-Habitat. Available at: https://mirror.unhabitat.org/list.asp?typeid=15&catid=559 (accessed 10 May 2021).

UN-Habitat (2008) *State of the World's Cities 2008/2009: Harmonious Cities*. Nairobi: UN-Habitat. Available at: https://unhabitat.org/state-of-the-worlds-cities-20082009-harmonious-cities-2 (accessed 12 May 2021).

UN-Habitat (2013) *State of Women in Cities 2012–2013: Gender and the Prosperity of Cities*. Nairobi: UN-Habitat,. Available at: https://unhabitat.org/gender-and-prosperity-of-cities-state-of-women-in-cities-20122013 (accessed 12 May 2021).

UN-Habitat (2020a) *Breaking Cycles of Risk Accumulation in African Cities*. Nairobi: UN-Habitat. Available at: https://unhabitat.org/breaking-cycles-of-risk-accumulation-in-african-cities (accessed 7 May 2021).

UN-Habitat (2020b) *World Cities Report 2020: The Value of Sustainable Urbanization*. Nairobi: UN-Habitat. Available at: https://unhabitat.org/World%20Cities%20Report%202020 (accessed 2 May 2021).

UNHCR (2018) *Global Trends: Forced Displacement in 2018*, United Nations High Commissioner for Refugees, Geneva. Available at: https://globalization.unhcr.org/5d08d7ee7.pdf (accessed 20 May 2021).

Wearesocial (2021) *Digital Report 2021*. Milan: Wearesocial. Available at: https://wearesocial.com/uk/blog/2021/04/60-percent-of-the-worlds-population-is-now-online (accessed 29 April 2021).

WHO (2008) *Closing the Gap in a Generation: Health Equity through Action on the Social Determinants of Health*. Final report of the commission on social determinants of health. Geneva: World Health Organization. Available at: https://globalization.who.int/social_determinants/final_report/csdh_finalreport_2008.pdf (accessed 1 May 2021).

WHO (2014) *Report of the Sage Working Group on Vaccine Hesitancy*. Geneva: World Health Organization. Available at: https://globalization.who.int/immunization/sage/meetings/2014/october/1_Report_WORKING_GROUP_vaccine_hesitancy_final.pdf (accessed 17 May 2021).

WHO (2019) *The Thirteenth General Programme of Work, 2019–2023*. Geneva: World Health Organization. Available at: https://globalization.who.int/about/what-we-do/thirteenth-general-programme-of-work-2019—2023 (accessed 16 May 2021).

WHO (2021) *Social Determinants of Health*. Geneva: World Health Organization. Available at: https://globalization.who.int/health-topics/social-determinants-of-health#tab=tab_1 (accessed 10 May 2021).

WHO and UN-Habitat (2010) *Hidden Cities: Unmasking and Overcoming Health Inequities in Urban Settings*. Geneva and Nairobi: WHO and UN-Habitat. Available at: https://globalization.who.int/publications/i/item/9789241548038 (accessed 10 April 2021).

WHO and UN-Habitat (2016) *Global Report on Urban Health: Equitable, Healthier Cities for Sustainable Development*. Geneva and Nairobi: WHO and UN-Habitat. Available at: https://apps.who.int/iris/handle/10665/204715 (accessed 22 April 2021).

Woods, M. (2017) Globalization and rural areas, *International Encyclopedia of Geography*, 2007: 1–6.

Zheng, Y., Ji, Y., Chang, C. et al. (2020) The evolution of health policy in China and internal migrants: continuity, change, and current implementation challenges, *Asia & the Pacific Policy Studies*, 7: 81–94.

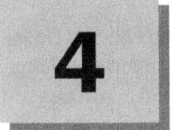

4

Emergence of global health governance

Preslava Stoeva

Overview

This chapter provides an historical perspective on key aspects of the emergence of global governance for public health. It outlines three main areas of continuity that connect the past to the present – regional and transregional governance cooperation to address threats to public health, the influence of colonialism on public health knowledge and practice, and the prominent role of private actors in shaping the architecture of global health governance.

Learning objectives

After working through this chapter, you will be able to:

- Describe the emergence of regional and transregional governance in historical perspective.
- Evaluate how and why patterns of global health governance have changed.
- Consider different historical influences on which contemporary global health challenges are addressed and how.

Key terms

Quarantine: A period and place of isolation in which people or animals arriving from another territory, or exposed to infectious or contagious disease, are placed.

Regional cooperation: Cooperation between states within the same geographic region. Regional cooperation between states tends to be more effective than international cooperation. States' geographic proximity, and the common challenges they face, are likely to intensify the need for cooperation and to make it more effective.

Trans-regional cooperation: Cooperation between states and organizations from different regions, defined by its focus on regional values and priorities.

Transboundary: Threats, concerns or issues that transcend national borders or have an influence that cannot be contained by such borders – e.g. viruses and pollution.

Colonial medicine and public health: Medical and public health knowledge developed in response to outbreaks of communicable diseases in territories under colonial control. Public health measures were developed to meet the needs of colonial settlers, soldiers and traders exposed to new communicable diseases with a view to facilitate administrative control; and to increase the economic productivity of colonialized peoples.

Regional and trans-regional cooperation for health

Early examples of regional cooperation to contain the transboundary spread of infectious diseases along trade and travel routes date back at least two centuries. It is worth acknowledging and understanding this history for three main reasons. First, cooperative efforts to address health-related threats (mainly infectious diseases) across different regions have a long and diverse history with early precedents of regional cooperation not entirely European-centric. Second and related to the first – states have demonstrated historical commitment to seeking collective solutions to problems associated with the transborder spread of diseases using different means: diplomatic conferences, international conventions and through inter-governmental organizations (at first regional and later international). Third, public health measures used to contain the spread of infectious diseases have not changed significantly over the centuries – quarantines and containment measures (e.g. restrictions on travel and trade) have most recently been introduced to manage the Covid-19 pandemic. These measures attract the same criticisms now as they did at the International Sanitary Conferences in the nineteenth century – that they disproportionately affect the economy, trade, travel and growth, along with scepticism regarding their effectiveness in stemming the spread of infection. As Liverani and Coker note, the 'history of these early efforts toward international cooperation is not only relevant as the background of current developments in international health... it also reflects wider issues of political culture and political economy' (2012: 918) (see also Chapter 5).

Early precedents of establishing national and regional health councils to facilitate regional cooperation for the protection of public health were based outside Europe. These include the Maritime et Quarantinaire d'Egypte, based in Alexandria (1831), Conseil Supérieur de Santé de Constantinople, Ottoman Empire (1839), the Conseil Sanitaire de Tanger, Morocco (1840) and the Conseil Sanitaire de Teheran set up by the Shah of Persia (1867). These councils included diplomatic representation from foreign powers (Howard-Jones 1950: 1034), demonstrating trans-regional reach. The Conseil Sanitaire d'Egypte later became the regional epidemiological bureau of the Office International d'Hygiène Publique (Lee 2009: 3). Meetings of these councils were irregular with a focus on containment and limiting the spread of infectious diseases through trade.

Regional cooperation on health in the late nineteenth century was emergent in the Americas as well. International sanitary conferences and meetings, involving the Brazilian Empire and the Republics of Uruguay, were held in Montevideo in 1873, in Rio de Janeiro in 1887 and in Lima, Peru, in 1888 (Chaves 2013: 1). As Chaves notes, the main objective of the conferences was 'the removal of obstacles to trade and transport and the protection of the region against what were seen as exotic epidemics' (2013: 3). While these objectives were similar to activities in other regions, the focus of activity was on preventing and containing yellow fever. The regulation of trade in order to maintain health was further discussed at the First International Conference of American States (1889–1890) (PAHO, n.d.). State leaders agreed to periodically hold health conventions and the Second International Conference of American States (1901–1902) recommended the establishment of a permanent executive board. The First International Sanitary Convention of the American Republics opened in 1902 and established the International Sanitary Bureau, headquartered in Washington, DC (PAHO, n.d.). The Bureau was later renamed the Pan-American Sanitary Bureau and is the predecessor of the Pan American Health Organization (PAHO), which is the oldest continually operating international health organization in the world.

Today PAHO serves as both the specialized health agency of the Inter-American system and the Regional Office for the Americas of the World Health Organization. Regional cooperation in the Americas was initiated to seek local solutions for local problems (PAHO, n.d.). The organization was small and worked with limited resources but laid the foundations of important future practices – such as transborder data collection, the exchange and sharing of information and independent regional health governance. There are three distinct characteristics of the early work of PAHO: the dominance of the United States in the organization in its early years; the desire to seek local solutions for local problems; and the introduction of the 'social medicine' approach, which emphasizes the social and economic determinants of specific population health problems (Waitzkin et al. 2001; Cueto 2006). These idiosyncrasies were generated in part by the specific political and economic realities in the Americas, but also by the socially focused politics of a number of Latin American states. The desire of the United States to play a leading role in regional and international cooperation (with a short relapse during the years of American isolationism in the 1930s and early 1940s) has not waned and has shaped various aspects of contemporary international politics for health – including a reliance on biomedical approaches, hegemonic leadership and pre-occupation with narrow American national and domestic interests. The leading role played by the United States in contemporary global public health can, therefore, be said to be a combination of US hegemonic ambitions and the continuation of colonial disease-eradication policy driven by economic interests, as discussed by Packard (2016). Kickbusch (2002) argues that analysts have not paid sufficient attention to the implications of the US leadership role in global public health and specifically to the ways in which the US has managed to dictate the global agenda in alignment with its narrow national interests.

The historiography of public health is still dominated by the work of European and North American historians and predominantly focused on regional cooperation in Europe and the United States (Fidler 2001). It is important to appreciate, however, that European cooperation in health was an integral part of a much longer and more diverse history of regional and trans-regional cooperation and that innovation and knowledge have been produced consistently across different regions. Fourteen International Sanitary Conferences (ISC) in total took place in Europe between 1851 and 1938. Four International Sanitary Conventions were agreed between 1892 and 1903. These were later consolidated into the International Sanitary Regulations – the predecessor of the International Health Regulations (Lee 2009: 3). Convened by the government of France, the conferences brought together diplomats from Europe and North America and sought to coordinate international efforts and establish agreed protective measures and standards on quarantine practices, so that these did not interfere with the growing volumes of international trade and travel (Howard-Jones 1975: 11).

Transborder cooperative efforts in Europe focused primarily on controlling the spread of three specific infectious diseases – the plague, cholera and yellow fever (Borowy 2010). The bubonic plague is believed to have spread to Europe from China, periodically causing epidemic outbreaks in Europe between 1347 and 1750 (Cockerham and Cockerham 2010: 43). Cholera – a disease endemic in India – caused a significant death toll in Europe in the nineteenth century (Liverani and Coker 2012: 917). Yellow fever is believed to have arrived in Europe through maritime trade routes with Africa and was then spread throughout the Northern hemisphere (Staples and Monath 2008).

Historically, states used different containment measures to prevent the spread of infectious diseases. These included closing ports (and cities) or keeping travellers and goods in quarantine. The lack of consensus and understanding of the causes of these infectious diseases hindered regional negotiations of solutions. In 1907, the Office International d'Hygiène Publique (OIHP) was established in Paris to collect and share information and epidemiological data on cholera, the plague and yellow fever. The OIHP has since been incorporated in the administrative mechanisms of the World Health Organization (WHO), which is now a focal point for the collection and sharing of epidemiological data on a very broad spectrum of diseases across the world.

Decision-making on various aspects of public health continues to take place in the context of some regional organizations such as the European Union (EU), South American Economic Organization (MERCOSUR), Economic Community of West African States (ECOWAS) and the Association of South East Asian Nations (ASEAN), as well as through the regional offices of the WHO.

✎ **Activity 4.1**

What similarities and differences can you identify between historical examples of regional and transregional governance of health-related threats and contemporary approaches to global health governance? What are the key characteristics of global health governance that differentiate it from regional governance? Note down your reflections, then compare your ideas to the feedback below.

Feedback

In your response consider geographic focus – e.g. regional or international; think about whether there are organizational structures in place and whether these are permanent or ad hoc; consider what the mandate of different organizations is, what the focus of their activity is. While there are many similarities and therefore continuities, much has changed since the early days of regional governance of health threats. Howard-Jones (1950), for example, notes how the lack of medical knowledge of the causes of infectious diseases affected political decision-making on what the necessary steps were to prevent and contain these. Howard-Jones (1950) also notes the limited role played by medical professionals in the diplomatic negotiations – has this changed?

What these examples demonstrate is a recurring pattern of issue-specific, regional and transregional cooperation to gather information, share knowledge, seek resolution to collective problems and standardize responses crystallizing into more permanent inter-governmental organizations. This pattern of multilateral state-driven action has evolved but not changed significantly at its core; nineteenth century regional cooperation for health was shaped by the broader historic context within which it emerged. A defining characteristic of this context was the politics of colonial rule and empire-building, as discussed in the next section.

From tropical and colonial medicine to international health

As Europeans set off on journeys of geographic discovery in the fifteenth and sixteenth century, they established maritime trade routes and more frequent connections between what has been referred to as the 'Old World' (Eurasia and Africa) and the 'New World' (the Americas). The exchange of plants, animals and diseases promoted by these new connections are referred to as the 'Columbian exchange' (Crosby 1972), which forms part of biological globalization – defined as the global transfer and exchange of plants, animals and diseases. The effects of the Columbian exchange – particularly the transfer of infectious diseases from Eurasia, e.g. measles, smallpox, influenza, mumps, typhus, whooping cough, as well as malaria and yellow fever from Africa – had catastrophic consequences for the indigenous populations (Montenegro and Stephens 2007). The scale of impact of these diseases on indigenous populations is only partially understood, due to the lack of data on population size. Historians have tried to compensate for this lack of data by constructing estimates of indigenous population numbers and patterns of morbidity and mortality among these populations before and after the European invasion (McNeill 1976). This part of the Columbian exchange was mostly one-directional, flowing from the Old World to the New World.

It is in this broader historic context of trans-continental travel, trade and conquest that we begin to see the effects of continuous trans-regional spread of infectious disease on population health and the emergent need for regional and transregional sanitary cooperation as discussed previously. A specific branch of medicine began to emerge to respond to the threats posed by 'tropical' diseases to European merchants, soldiers and sailors (Arnold 1997). The relationship between tropical and colonial medicine is contested – while the terms are often used interchangeably, some authors draw a distinction between them. Thus, Warren (1990) uses historical sources to demonstrate that tropical medicine arose out of the needs of explorers and the military and later evolved 'as a necessary aspect of the colonial system' (Warren 1990: 143). The significance of Warren's distinction is that it draws attention to the diverse motivations in the establishment of these branches of public health and could explain differences in focus between tropical and colonial medicine. The term tropical medicine continues to be used, and both the Liverpool and London Schools still use 'tropical medicine' in their names, but there have been calls for the field to be subsumed into more relevant broader fields – e.g. infectious diseases, travel medicine and economic studies of health systems (De Cock et al. 1995).

With the spread of colonial conquest and colonial extraction of raw materials in the eighteenth and nineteenth century, the needs of imperial powers for epidemiologic knowledge associated with colonial settlement and exploitation gave rise to the emerging field of colonial medicine. As

European states and later the United States expanded colonial subjugation, extraction and enslavement to territories in Africa, South America and the Caribbean, imperial soldiers, settlers and officials came into contact with unfamiliar and deadly infectious diseases. Morbidity and mortality among colonial subjects impacted economic productivity and rates of extraction, which affected colonial interests.

Key features of colonial public health campaigns can be said to constitute examples of continuity, connecting colonial health with international and global health. As Randall argues, colonial health campaigns were driven by the interests of colonial powers, designed outside the countries where the health problems were located, and often imposed by force (or threat of legal action), against the will of and without (or with little) consultation with the local population (Packard 2016: 8). Packard describes campaigns in Cuba, Panama and the Philippines to eradicate yellow fever, which he notes are consistent in their approach with methods used by European colonial authorities in Africa and South Asia to tackle cholera, plague, sleeping sickness and malaria (2016: 19–22). Colonial medical campaigns were often disease-specific and did not contribute to the development of local health systems. Campaigns predominantly adopted a biomedical approach, utilizing various technologies to address health problems, with some exceptions where changes to living conditions of workers were recommended, recognizing the influence of broader determinants of health. The preference for biomedical knowledge and technologies often devalued local and indigenous knowledge, contributing to the broader sense of the superiority of colonial powers, thus generating and re-enforcing a dependency between colonized states and colonial powers. The significance of indigenous knowledge and the rights of indigenous people, including their right to health, to participation in determining their health programmes and their right to traditional medicines are recognized and re-affirmed by the United Nations Permanent Forum on Indigenous Issues, established in 2000, and in the annual reports the forum produces: 'State of the World's Indigenous Peoples' (UNFPII, n.d.).

Another aspect of colonialism is the appropriation of indigenous knowledge, local and regional practice, along with the limited recognition of local innovation and resistance to colonial imposition. Striking examples of extraction and appropriation not only of resources and raw materials but also of indigenous knowledge are presented in Espinosa's (2013) study advocating a global approach to the history of disease, medicine and public health, which recognizes the contributions emerging from Latin America. Espinosa draws on existing Latin American historiography describing the role of indigenous knowledge as a source of medicines – including the synthesis of diosgenin for the production of synthetic hormones and other medicines from wild yam grown in Mexico or the discovery by Jesuit priests of the medicinal qualities of cinchona bark – a source of quinine – in Peru (2013: 802–803). She highlights the contribution of a Cuban doctor – Carlos

Finlay – to identifying the cause of yellow fever and of a Colombian doctor – Roberto Franco – in identifying the dual cycles of transmission of yellow fever between mosquitoes in urban and jungle areas, which were affecting the success of urban campaigns to eradicate the disease (Espinosa 2013: 803–805). The knowledge contributions of both of these doctors were obscured and appropriated by colonial authorities. What these examples further illustrate is the interconnectedness and entanglements of developments in public health knowledge and practice across different parts of the world, but also that flows of knowledge and ideas were never one-way from core to periphery.

The fields of tropical and colonial medicine were implicated in the emergence of the public health subfield of international health. International health focuses on similar concerns – i.e. diseases specific to low- and middle-income settings, health promotion and development but further reflects on the involvement of inter-governmental organizations like WHO and private actors such as philanthropic foundations like the Rockefeller Foundation (to which we will return in the next section) in the search for solutions to these concerns. Brown et al. (2006) further put the WHO and its historical transformation at the heart of the transition from the terminology of 'international health' to the then emerging concept of global health, to situate these developments in a historical context, which also serves to demonstrate their interconnectedness. In other words, one could argue that the contemporary concept of 'global health' is rooted in tropical and colonial medicine and knowledge, which further explains why continuities, such as classifying diseases as 'tropical', or designing interventions and using a biomedical approach to addressing such diseases and their causes, require critical attention, as they reverberate through history to the present (Fofana 2020: 2–6; Holst 2020: 3). In particular, behind the medical knowledge associated with diseases specific to particular geographic regions, there are more sinister practices stemming from tropical and colonial medicine associated, for example, with constructions of race, 'othering', marginalization, assumptions of civilization, superiority and supremacy, which represent fundamental aspects of social and political relations and power inequalities between imperial centres and their colonies, and which are perpetuating discrimination and inequalities long after political decolonization has taken place (Dionne and Turkmen 2020). As Cueto et al. argue, acknowledging the research and history of global health – 'tracing cross-national connections and entanglements, giving due attention to developments in colonial and postcolonial spaces, exploring the construction of asymmetric hierarchical networks and examining how people, ideas and practices have changed in processes of transnational circulation' can help us better understand local, national and international contemporary global health challenges (2020: 7).

Analysts have observed that the global response to the Covid-19 pandemic has displayed characteristics consistent with historical patterns of coloniality, discrimination and marginalization. As Bump et al. point out, 'morbidity and mortality are far worse for indigenous people, migrants, black people, and other victims of racism, discrimination and marginalization' (2021: 1). Responses to the pandemic exhibit resemblances to colonial medicine – illustrated, for example, by nationalistic competition for resources such as excessive procurement of personal protective equipment and vaccines; excessive emphasis on diseases and biomedical factors; side-lining social and economic determinants of health; emphasis on knowledge flowing from north to south; presumptions that approaches to containing the pandemic in African countries will fail; exploitative attitudes hindering global collective, collaborative, approaches to containing the pandemic and reducing its negative effects on the most vulnerable (Bump et al. 2021; also Dionne and Turkmen 2020; Fofana 2020). Since these have been identified not only as recurring patterns of colonial medicine, but also significant shortcomings in the global response to Covid-19, there is both ethical and practical value in critically examining persistent coloniality. Despite the near completion of the political process of decolonization in the 1960s and 1970s, the UN decolonization programme continues to exist, as 17 Non-Self-Governing Territories, home to nearly 2 million people, have still not achieved self-determination through independence, free association or integration with an independent state (United Nations, n.d.).

Analysts have called for the recognition of the impact of colonial legacies and the need to reform global health and pandemic response towards more inclusivity, power and resource redistribution and sharing. Steps that are considered key in this process include grounding global health policy in health justice and equity frameworks, upholding human rights, 'abrogat[ing] structures that perpetuate exploitation and dispossession', generating awareness and response to structural violence and structural vulnerability (Büyüm et al. 2020; Fofana 2020). The Covid-19 pandemic and the observed weaknesses of global, regional and local governance may provide a significant catalyst and an opportunity for more profound changes to the global system that can make it fairer and more effective for all.

✏ Activity 4.2

Think about a contemporary health issue that you are familiar with through research, work or study. Can you identify elements of colonial medicine (or the assumptions, approaches and practices that characterize colonial medicine) in the ways in which the issue is framed and/or addressed? Note down your reflections in light of the discussion above, then compare your ideas to the feedback below.

Feedback

Colonial medicine has distinct characteristics as discussed above, which have travelled through time and practice. Aspects of coloniality can be detected in public health campaigns, in research, in programmes to address specific diseases. Legacies of colonial medicine include interventionist public health, narrow focus on acute health crises, investment in isolated campaigns, but no investment in strengthening health systems, perpetuating health inequities, and paying limited attention to the socio-economic determinants of health. Are any of these identifiable in relation to the health issue that you have chosen? Can you think of other colonial medicine legacies?

Non-state actors in international health

In addition to early inter-governmental cooperation, there is a history over a century old of non-state and private actors' involvement in health, raising questions about the purpose and nature of their involvement, role and contribution to a field generally governed by public authority. Tensions between public authority and private action and resources, and also the relationship between these raise questions about transparency, accountability, legitimacy and ethics. These are further discussed in Chapter 12. The discussion below briefly presents the historic involvement of non-state actors in public health as a way of illustrating both different ways in which these actors have been involved but also their embeddedness in the global health governance system.

One of the most recognizable global private organizations – the International Red Cross and Red Crescent Movement (ICRC) – started in 1863 as the International Committee to Aid the Military Wounded, by a group of five individuals: Henry Dunant, a Swiss banker, Gustave Moynier, a Swiss lawyer, General Dufour, commander of the Swiss Army, and two physicians, Louis Appia and Theodore Maunoir. They were determined to create national relief societies, staffed by qualified volunteers to care for the wounded in wartime. The organization's initial scope of activity – assisting wounded soldiers in international war – has expanded to cover various aspects of humanitarian work – helping civilians, refugees and internally displaced persons, etc. (Forsythe 2005: 2). The ICRC's mission is to 'alleviate human suffering, protect life and health, and uphold human dignity especially during armed conflicts and other emergencies' (ICRC 2021). The movement works closely with other non-governmental organizations and is funded largely by voluntary donations from national governments and individuals. The ICRC is, on the one hand, a unique type of organization due to its development, main characteristics and unusual relationship with national governments (Forsythe 2005), but, on the other, a typical example of a global private actor, unregulated by governments, which delivers healthcare services and humanitarian assistance, in tandem with other NGOs such as Médecins Sans Frontières (MSF) and Oxfam, and strives to abide by the humanitarian principles of humanity, impartiality, neutrality and independence.

The beginning of the twentieth century saw the emergence of another very particular type of non-governmental entity – the philanthropic foundation. The Rockefeller Foundation was one of a number of private funds and foundations (including the Carnegie Foundation, Milbank Memorial Fund and Sage Foundation), which provided finance for education, health and biomedical research, both domestically in the United States and abroad. These include establishing training centres, schools of public health, education and research programmes in Europe (Weindling 1993), the Far East and Latin America (Weindling 1995; Cueto 1997). The Rockefeller Sanitary Commission for the Eradication of Hookworm Disease was established in 1909 to address hookworm disease in the southern states of the United States, where the Rockefellers had direct economic interests in the production of raw materials (Brown 1976: 898). Brown's research has drawn on information collected from the archives of the Foundation, including internal memos, correspondence and reports to highlight the intentions behind health-related investments to conclude that the aim of the Foundation's programmes was 'to raise the productivity of the workers in underdeveloped countries . . . to reduce the cultural autonomy of these agrarian peoples . . . [and] to assuage hostility to the US and undermine goals of national economic and political independence' (Brown 1976: 900). Birn and Fee similarly observed that through its leadership in the hookworm, yellow fever and malaria campaigns, the Rockefeller Foundation prepared vast regions for investment and increased productivity.

Additionally, the Rockefeller Foundation was directly involved in the appropriation of local knowledge and expertise in Latin America, which adds another layer to the deeply embedded coloniality of its activities (Espinosa 2013). It chose its interventions carefully to avoid campaigns that would be 'costly, overly complex, time-consuming, or distracting to its technically oriented public health model and its focused means of measuring success' (Birn and Fee 2013: 1618) – a common feature of many contemporary interventions, which select 'easy wins' over longer term work to support the development of sustainable and resilient health systems. In reflecting on historic accounts of Rockefeller campaigns in Latin America, however, Espinosa (2013) argues that the Foundation was rarely able to impose health reforms in the region and that its programmes were only successful when they were negotiated with local actors. This is an important observation, as it counters conventional views of Latin America as a passive receiver of colonial interventions. Resistance and contestation are important forces in political spaces.

The Rockefeller Foundation further provided considerable financial support to the League of Nations Health Organization and is credited with
inventing the public–private partnership model, which is now common in
global health. The work of the Foundation helped establish a technically
oriented approach to health emulated by other foundations, including the
Bill and Melinda Gates Foundation.

✎ Activity 4.3

Thinking about the Covid-19 pandemic, what historical continuities can
you identify? What has changed from the early examples of communicable diseases of pandemic potential?

Feedback

In many ways, the public health response to the Covid-19 pandemic
resembles public health measures taken by governments centuries
ago – using quarantine measures, restricting travel, identifying and doc-
umenting cases, sharing epidemiological information nationally and
internationally. Medical knowledge and technology, however, is very different to that in previous centuries, so the ways in which these practices
are undertaken has evolved in response to this. For example, identifying
Covid-19 cases, and alerting those in close contact with them can be
done via smart phone apps, but the logic of the process remains very
similar to the pre-digital era. The DNA of the virus was isolated quickly,
allowing vaccines to reduce transmission and acute illness to be developed. Governments engaged with experts in search of effective solutions to the prevention of transmission and containment of the pandemic.
International organizations attempted to coordinate national and global
responses, albeit faced with many of the challenges which these bodies
face in the arena of international politics, in health and beyond (see
Chapters 9 and 10).

Summary

This chapter explored the history of international and global cooperative
efforts to respond to transborder health challenges and sketched some
aspects of the historical foundations of contemporary global health governance. There are notable themes in these early efforts for transborder
cooperation on issues of population health. Some of the patterns of engagement and activity – such as those exhibited in regional cooperation – were

consensual, cooperative and driven by common interests among equal partners. These crystallized in the establishment of regional inter-governmental organizations and the creation of international treaties – such as the International Sanitary Conventions. Other patterns of engagement, however, were oppressive, intrusive, premised on assumptions about the inferiority of indigenous populations. Relationships of unequal power are often very visible. They define the nature of political relations among actors globally and pervade intergovernmental organizations and decision-making processes. The politics of colonial extraction and oppression have had a profound influence on shaping the field of global health governance, as well as the ways health priorities are set and health initiatives delivered. Taking a historical perspective allows us to examine the extent to which continuities persist and shape contemporary governance of health, which is further explored in the following chapters.

References

Arnold, D. (1997) The place of 'the Tropics' in Western medical ideas since 1750, *Tropical Medicine & International Health*, 2(4): 303–313.

Birn, A. and Fee, E. (2013) The Rockefeller Foundation and the international health agenda, *The Lancet*, 381 (9878): 1618– 1619.

Borowy, I. (2010) The League of Nations Health Organisation: from European to global health governance?, in A. Andresen, W. Hubbard and T. Ryymin (eds) *International and Local Approaches to Health and Health Care*. Bergen: University of Bergen.

Brown, E.R. (1976) Public health in imperialism: early Rockefeller programs at home and abroad, *American Journal of Public Health*, 66: 897–903.

Brown, T., Cueto, M. and Fee, E. (2006) The World Health Organization and the transition from 'international' to 'global' public health, *American Journal of Public Health*, 96(1): 62–72.

Bump, J.B., Baum, F., Sakornsin, M. et al. (2021) Political economy of Covid-19: extractive, regressive, competitive, *BMJ*, 372: n73.

Büyüm, A., Kenney, C., Koris, A. et al. (2020) Decolonising global health: if not now, when?, *BMJ Global Health*, 5(8): e003394.

Chaves, C. (2013) Power and health in South America: international sanitary conferences, 1870–1889, *História, Ciências, Saúde-Manguinhos*, 20: 411–434.

Cockerham, G. and Cockerham, W. (2010) *Health and Globalization*. Cambridge: Polity Press.

Crosby Jr, A. (1972) *The Columbian Exchange: Biological and Cultural Consequences of 1492*, 30th edn. Westport, CT: Praeger.

Cueto, M. (1997) Science under adversity: Latin American medical research and American private philanthropy, 1920–1960, *Minerva*, 35: 233–245.

Cueto, M. (2006) *The Value of Health: A History of the Pan American Health Organization*. Washington, DC: PAHO. Available at: https://iris.paho.org/handle/10665.2/51500 (accessed 22 June 2021).

Cueto, M., Rodogno, D. and Bourbonnais, N. (2020) The meaning(s) of global public health history, *História, Ciências, Saúde-Manguinhos*, 27(1): 7–10.

De Cock, K.M., Lucas, S., Mabey, D. et al. (1995) Tropical medicine for the 21st century, *BMJ (Clinical Research Ed.)*, 311(7009): 860–862.

Dionne, K. and Turkmen, F. (2020) The politics of pandemic othering: putting Covid-19 in global and historical context, *International Organization*, 74(S1): E213–E230.

Espinosa, M. (2013) Globalizing the history of disease, medicine, and public health in Latin America, *Isis*, 104(4): 798–806.

Fidler, D. (2001) The globalization of public health: the first 100 years of international health diplomacy, *Bulletin of the World Health Organization*, 79(9): 842–849.

Fofana, M. (2020) Decolonising global health in the time of Covid-1, *Global Public Health*, 16(8–9): 1155–1166.

Forsythe, D. (2005) *The Humanitarians: The International Committee of the Red Cross*. Cambridge: Cambridge University Press.

Holst, J. (2020) Global health – emergence, hegemonic trends and biomedical reductionism, *Globalization and Health*, 16(42). https://doi.org/10.1186/s12992-020-00573-4.

Howard-Jones, N. (1950) Origins of international health work, *British Medical Journal*, 1(4661): 1032–1037.

Howard-Jones, N. (1975) *The Scientific Background of the International Sanitary Conferences, 1851–1938*. Geneva: World Health Organization. Available at: https://apps.who.int/iris/handle/10665/62873 (accessed 21 June 2021)

ICRC (2021) *The International Red Cross and Red Crescent Movement*. Geneva: ICRC. Available at: https://globalization.icrc.org/en/who-we-are/movement (accessed 13 June 2021).

Kickbusch, I. (2002) Influence and opportunity: reflections on the US role in global public health, *Health Affairs*, 21(6): 131–141.

Lee, K. (2009) *The World Health Organization (WHO)*. London: Routledge.

Liverani, M. and Coker, R. (2012) Protecting Europe from diseases: from the International Sanitary Conferences to the ECDC, *Journal of Health Politics, Policy and Law*, 37: 915–934.

Pan American Health Organization (PAHO) (n.d.) History of PAHO. Available at: https://globalization.paho.org/en/who-we-are/history-paho (accessed 22 June 2021).

McNeill, W.H. (1976) *Plagues and Peoples*. London: Penguin Books.

Montenegro, R.A. and Stephens, C. (2006) Indigenous health in Latin America and the Caribbean, *Lancet*, 367(9525): 1859–1869.

Packard, R. (2016) *A History of Global Health – Interventions into the Lives of Other Peoples*. Baltimore, MD: Johns Hopkins University Press.

Staples, J. and Monath, T. (2008) Yellow fever: 100 years of discovery, *JAMA*, 300(8): 960.

United Nations (n.d.) The United Nations and decolonization. Available at: https://globalization.un.org/dppa/decolonization/en (accessed 22 June 2021).

United Nations Permanent Forum for Indigenous Issues (UNFPII) (n.d.). Available at: https://globalization.un.org/development/desa/indigenouspeoples/ (accessed 23 June 2021).

Waitzkin, H., Iriart, C., Estrada, A. et al. (2001) Social medicine then and now: lessons from Latin America, *American Journal of Public Health*, 91(10): 1592–1601.

Warren, K. (1990) Tropical medicine or tropical health: the Heath Clark lectures, 1988, *Reviews of Infectious Diseases*, 12(1): 142–156.

Weindling, P. (1993) Public health and political stabilisation: the Rockefeller Foundation in Central and Eastern Europe between the two World Wars, *Minerva*, 31: 253–267.

Weindling, P. (ed.) (1995) *International Health Organisations and Movements, 1918–1939*. Cambridge: Cambridge University Press.

PART 2

Critical issues in global health

Globalization and infectious diseases

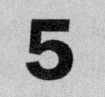

5

Marco Liverani

Overview

After centuries of recurring and devastating epidemics, during the 1970s there was a widespread belief that infectious diseases would soon become a thing of the past. From the 1980s to the present, however, the emergence and global spread of HIV/AIDS, SARS, Ebola, antimicrobial resistance and the Covid-19 pandemic, alongside the resurgence of diseases such as malaria, have been painful reminders that infectious diseases still have the potential to cause death, poverty and suffering on a global scale. The first part of this chapter explores links between these challenges and globalization, with particular attention to the role of human mobility, changes in food production systems and economic inequalities. In the second part, we consider the institutions and mechanisms established to address these shared health threats, from early developments in the nineteenth century to the present framework of global disease surveillance.

Learning objectives

After working through this chapter, you will be able to:

- Critically assess ways in which processes of globalization have the potential to increase or reduce the risk of disease emergence and transmission.
- Evaluate mechanisms of international cooperation for infectious diseases prevention and control within their historical background.
- Identify elements of change, continuity and key challenges in the present context of global disease surveillance and response.

Key terms

Antimicrobial resistance: A phenomenon that occurs when microorganisms – such as bacteria, viruses, fungi and parasites – change over time and no longer respond to medicines that are used to treat them. As a result, antibiotics and other antimicrobial medicines become less effective, increasing the risk of disease spread, severe illness and death.

Emerging infectious diseases: Diseases that have appeared in a population for the first time or that may have existed previously but are rapidly increasing in incidence or geographic range.

International Health Regulations: An international instrument that is legally binding on all WHO member states and aims to protect against the international spread of disease, avoiding unnecessary interference with international traffic and trade.

Pandemic: An epidemic occurring worldwide, or over a very wide area, usually affecting a large number of people.

Globalization and infectious disease risk

Over the past century, global patterns of disease and mortality have changed. Thanks to improved healthcare, sanitation, vaccines and antibiotics, infectious diseases are no longer the leading cause of death globally. As further discussed in Chapter 6, many countries have experienced an 'epidemiological transition' to a higher burden of non-communicable diseases. Nonetheless, infectious diseases remain an important global health concern. First, the epidemiological transition has been more pronounced in wealthy, industrialized countries; in low-income countries, a transition is also apparent, but respiratory infections and other communicable diseases such as malaria, HIV and TB are still a top cause of death (WHO 2020). Second, even in high-income countries, infectious diseases never really went away and have still the potential to cause major global health and economic crises as illustrated by the impact of HIV/AIDS, SARS and Covid-19. In 2020 alone, the Covid-19 pandemic caused more than 2 million deaths and an estimated cost to the global economy of US$11.7 trillion (Marcos Barba et al. 2020), taking a huge toll in the US and European countries. Furthermore, there are great global concerns about increasing antimicrobial resistance, which occurs when pathogens change over time and no longer respond to medicines that used to treat them, including antibiotics. If appropriate measures are not taken, it is predicted that drug resistant infections will cause 10 million deaths annually by 2050, particularly in low- and middle-income countries (LMICs) where the burden of infectious diseases is higher (O'Neill 2014).

The links between these trends and globalization are multidimensional. Globalization is a process involving social, economic and cultural developments that have created new connections and interdependencies between people, places and environments (see Chapter 1). As such, it can influence in multiple ways whether a pathogen survives, evolves, infects susceptible hosts and spreads widely (Saker et al. 2007). In the following sections, we will examine some of these developments and their direct or indirect role in disease emergence and transmission.

Population mobility

Population movements have been a source of disease transmission throughout human history as microbes have always travelled with human carriers and other vectors along trade, migratory and military routes. In the fourteenth century, the bubonic plague (known as the Black Death) entered Europe via Italy, carried by rats on Genoese trading ships sailing from the Black Sea, eventually killing almost one-third of Europe's population. In the past 200 years, progress in public health and medicine has been remarkable; however, the intensification of travel and commerce has provided new opportunities for the rapid transmission of diseases across countries and continents. An early example is the spread of cholera in the nineteenth century (Figure 5.1), which swept the globe in repeated waves along increasingly interconnected trade routes, from India to China and from Europe to the United States. In 1832, a British journalist noted that cholera 'mastered every variety of climate, surmounted every natural obstacle,

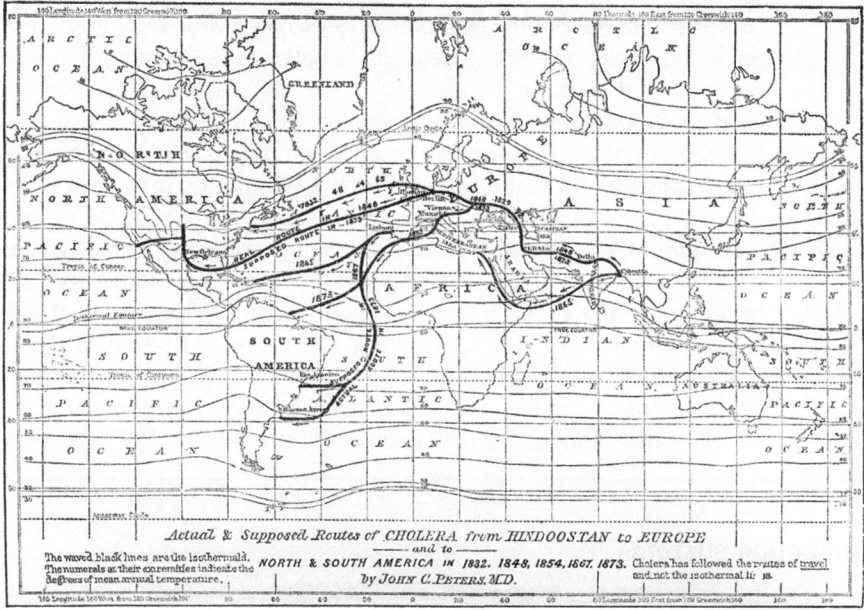

Figure 5.1: 'Actual and supposed routes of cholera from Hindoostan to Europe and North America in 1832, 1848, 1854, 1867 and 1873', from *A Treatise on Asiatic Cholera*, edited and prepared by Edmund Charles Wendt in association with John C. Peters, 1885

conquered every people' (in Briggs 1961: 76). Towards the end of the century, the term 'pandemic' (from Greek *pandēmos*, 'all people') became a household word to indicate a highly contagious disease which spreads rapidly across large geographic areas (Morens et al. 2009).

From the end of the Second World War to the present, the international flow of people and goods further increased due to leisure and business travel, trade liberalization, labour migration and increasing affordability of long-distance travel. In 1970, there were only about 9 million departures of registered air carriers worldwide but in 2019 the number exceeded 37 million (Figure 5.2). In 2018, the International Civil Aviation Organization (ICAO) reported that the total number of passengers carried on scheduled services in one year was 4.3 billion and was estimated to increase to 6.4 billion in 2030 (ICAO 2018). As described in Box 5.1, the rapid spread of SARS in 2003 exemplifies the public health implications of these trends. Air transport also played a key role in the early progression of the Covid-19 pandemic. After its origin in Wuhan, China, in December 2019, the disease reached virtually every country in the world by mid-2020 except for a handful of nations – most of them remote islands in the Pacific.

Box 5.1   The international spread of SARS

Severe acute respiratory syndrome (SARS) is a viral respiratory disease of zoonotic origin, which is believed to have crossed the barrier between animals and humans only recently. The first case of SARS was identified in Guangdong Province, China, in November 2002. The disease spread out of Guangdong Province in February 2003, when an infected physician spent a night in a hotel in the Hong Kong district of Kowloon, one of the most densely populated areas in the world. By the end of February, the disease was carried along major air travel routes as guests who had stayed at the same hotel flew home to Canada, Singapore, and other countries. As of August 2003, when the World Health Organization (WHO) declared the world SARS-free, the disease had spread to 29 countries, resulting in 8096 probable cases and 774 deaths worldwide, and significant social and economic impacts in areas with sustained transmission.

Food production systems

Most human infections have animal origins and have been linked with food production systems since the dawn of civilization. Domestication of wild animals brought them into closer contact with human populations, resulting in greater opportunities for disease emergence and rapid human-to-human transmission in larger and more crowded settlements and cities

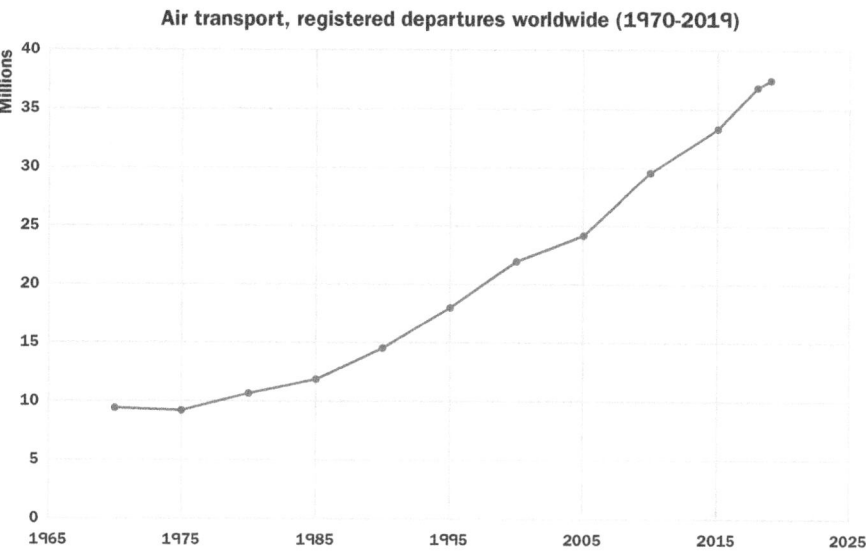

Figure 5.2: Registered air departures worldwide
Source: Chart produced using World Bank data

(Diamond 2002). As Chapter 3 discussed, with subsequent industrializa-tion and urbanization, consumers became separated from livestock production, creating diverse wildlife–livestock–human interfaces. At the same time, new methods of livestock production were developed to increase outputs and reduce costs, characterized by the confinement of large numbers of animals in housing units, use of concentrate feed, reduced genetic diversity and industrial management practices. This 'land-less' mode of production emerged in the United Kingdom and the United States in the 1930s (Woods 2012) and is increasingly common in many LMICs, particularly in the poultry and pig sectors (Robinson 2011). As Chapter 7 discusses, in the future, this trend towards intensified produc-tion is predicted to accelerate as a result of population growth (the global population will reach an estimated 10 billion by 2050) and income growth in LMICs, requiring commensurate shifts in output and land-use changes to meet increasing demand for meat products (FAO 2017).

While intensified production units are typically well isolated from contact with external sources of pathogens, their capacity to spread disease is still considerable, through high density of susceptible animals in communal housing, through the intensive movement of stock and feed, and through the international markets that they supply (Liverani et al. 2013). Further-more, the scale of livestock production is increasingly transnational, moving diseases rapidly across countries, as seen in the outbreaks of highly pathogenic avian influenza H5N1 and variants (Pfeiffer et al. 2011). Similar trends can be observed in food-borne infections caused by contaminated fruits, vegetables, milk products and other products. In 2007, an international outbreak of salmonella infection, linked to contaminated basil from Israel, affected individuals from England, Wales, Scotland, Denmark, the Netherlands and the USA (Elviss et al. 2009). Man-made interventions associated with food production also alter fundamental ecosystems and the geographical distribution of human populations and animal species, with mixed effects that may increase or reduce infectious disease risk (Fornace et al. 2013). For example, deforestation has reduced the natural habitat of the main malaria vector in Southeast Asia, the *Anopheles dirus* mosquito, which depends on deep forest shade for breeding; in other regions, however, forest clearing for farming has increased the abundance of malaria vectors that benefit from open landscapes for their larval habitats such as the *A. darlingi* mosquito in South America (Vittor et al. 2009; Laporta et al. 2021).

Global inequalities

As discussed in Chapters 2 and 3, socio-economic change and unequal access to resources, including healthcare, are other key factors that can affect infectious disease risk. Globalization has brought benefits, wealth and opportunities to some people but has also created or reinforced inequalities, leaving many others vulnerable to disease and deprivation. It is now clear, for example, that the abrupt transition of Russia to global capitalism after the dissolution of the Soviet Union in 1991 and the resulting collapse of the health system largely contributed to the resurgence of tuberculosis among impoverished population groups in this country, while the incomplete antibiotic courses many patients received has been a key driver of antibiotic resistance (Coker et al. 2008). The outbreaks of Ebola in Western Africa between 2013 and 2016 also highlighted profound global inequities and how these can interact with other factors in complex causal mechanisms to create high-risk environments (see Box 5.2). Beyond the number of cases, the outbreak also had a considerable socio-economic impact on the lives of those who were not affected directly, through the indirect consequences of disruptions to routine healthcare, school closure, loss of income and food insecurity. Thus, similar to non-communicable diseases (see Chapter 6), poverty, globalization and infectious diseases are linked in complex, non-linear ways. Impoverished population groups are more vulnerable to infections as a result of inadequate access to healthcare and medicines, malnutrition and poor sanitation. In turn, protracted ill health reduces work capacity and productivity, aggravating poverty and inequities. These links are well documented in the case of HIV/AIDS – defined by Barnett and Whitehead (2002) as 'the first epidemic of globalization' – which has been a major threat to development, economic growth and poverty alleviation in Africa for several decades.

Box 5.2 The Ebola epidemic

The first documented case in the 2013–2016 Ebola epidemic was Emile Ouamouno, a two-year-old boy in a village located in the Forest Region of Guinea. Despite its name, this region has suffered extensive deforestation due to mining and logging operations – a process that has brought wild animals, and particularly the Angolan bat species, which is thought to be the natural reservoir of the Ebola virus, into closer contact with human settlements. In December 2013, Emile developed severe illness after playing in the vicinity of a hollow tree housing a colony of bats and died. In January 2014, members of his family developed similar symptoms, followed by rapid death. In the following weeks, the virus spread to Conakry, Guinea's capital, and then to Liberia and Sierra Leone via cross-border movements of poor people looking for work or food. As the situation improved in one country, that country attracted patients from neighbouring countries seeking free hospital beds, thus reactivating transmission chains. By the end of 2014, the disease had spread widely throughout West Africa as a result of weak health systems, poor coordination between health authorities, mistrust in governments and Western medicine, and burial practices involving contact with Ebola-infected corpses – a combination that created a 'perfect storm' of disease risk and public health challenges (Piot 2014). The virus eventually found its way into Europe and the USA. Countries with greater resources and stronger health systems were able to control the disease more quickly and reported only a few cases.

✐ **Activity 5.1**

Antibiotics have revolutionized modern medicine in many respects, saving countless lives. However, increasing use of antibiotics for human and animal health since their introduction around 1950 has contributed to the evolution of antibiotic-resistant bacteria. As a result, in many regions some critically important antibiotics are no longer effective in treating urinary tract infections, sepsis and some forms of diarrhoea. Can you identify ways in which globalization may drive the evolution and spread of resistant bacteria?

Feedback

Different dimensions of globalization are linked with antibiotic resistance. As we have seen, intensified livestock production is a central aspect of economic globalization, driven by increased demand for meat products and market competition. In such systems, antibiotics are often added to the animal feeds or drinking water in sub-therapeutic doses to help animals gain weight faster or to prevent diseases. These practices contribute to the emergence and evolution of resistant bacteria, including resistance to antibiotics that are critical for human health, while the global trade of meat products and international travel spread them far and wide. Excessive use of antibiotics for human health, promoted by the large availability of antibiotics at low cost through global supply chains, is another key driver of increasing resistance. In developing countries, inadequate access to healthcare, unregulated dispensing and manufacture of antimicrobials, and inappropriate use further contribute to the development of drug-resistant organisms.

The globalization of infectious disease prevention and control

As discussed in Chapter 3, globalizing processes have increased mobility of people and goods. This has created new opportunities for the emergence and transnational spread of disease. At the same time, as discussed in Chapter 4, the intensification of international relations has led to the establishment of new institutional frameworks and cooperative arrangements to respond to these challenges.

From the International Sanitary Conferences to the WHO

As described in Chapter 4, early developments date back to the mid-nineteenth century, when national authorities began to attend the International Sanitary Conferences and discuss standard regulations and procedures against the spread of diseases. After several failed attempts, the first International Sanitary Convention was finally approved in 1892, to establish quarantine regulations for ships travelling through the Suez Canal. Opened in 1861, the canal was a key transportation route for international trade. However, medical administrators were concerned that the canal might be a channel for the spread in Europe of health threats that were perceived to originate in Asia and the Middle East. Similar concerns about the need to protect the European space from 'Asiatic diseases' were reflected in subsequent sanitary agreements, such as those regulating the flow of people during the annual Mecca pilgrimage (Huber 2006).

In the following decades, international conferences became a regular forum for health authorities and researchers, leading to the adoption of additional treaties on specific public health issues. Subsequent developments included the establishment of the Pan-American Sanitary Bureau in Washington, DC in 1896 and the Office International d'Hygiène Publique

(OIHP) in Paris in 1907, which were responsible for gathering information related to infectious disease outbreaks (see Chapter 4). Of particular importance was the public health work of the League of Nations (1919), whose administrative structure with three bodies (General Advisory Health Council, Health Committee and Secretariat) was a precursor to the World Health Organization (WHO). While the primary aim of the League of Nations was the promotion of collective security and the peaceful resolution of conflicts, member states were also required to take steps in matters of international concern for the prevention and control of disease, including sharing of epidemiological data and the standardization of biological products.

At the end of the Second World War, these pioneering efforts in international health cooperation were carried on by the United Nations and its health agency, the WHO. Established in 1948, the WHO incorporated into a single body the former international health offices and was given the mandate to unify the patchwork of ad-hoc sanitary conventions into a single set of binding rules on quarantine requirements, called the International Sanitary Regulations (ISR). Under the ISR (1951), WHO member states were mandated to notify outbreaks of 'quarantinable' diseases (plague, cholera, smallpox, yellow fever, typhus and relapsing fever) and to provide supplementary information on 'the source and type of the disease, the number of cases and deaths, the conditions affecting the spread of the diseases, and the prophylactic measures taken' (WHO 1951).

Similar to the concerns of the early sanitary conventions, these rules reflected a tension between public health needs and the imperative of global trade, exemplified in the mandate to 'ensure the maximum security against the international spread of disease with the minimum interference with world traffic' (WHO 1951). Yet the new regime of international health cooperation was different in fundamental ways. Whereas previous interventions were shaped by the commercial interests of colonial powers and the need to protect the European space from external threats, the mandate of the WHO was supported by a universal vision of human health and well-being (Liverani and Coker 2012). Indeed, the preamble of the WHO Constitution (1948) states that 'the enjoyment of the highest attainable standard of health is one of the fundamental rights of every human being without distinction of race, religion, political belief, economic or social condition' (WHO 1948). Furthermore, the new legal framework granted equal sovereign rights to newly independent states and former colonial powers. While colonial administrators oversaw and controlled the report of disease outbreaks through dedicated offices (such as the Far Eastern Bureau of the League of Nations, located in Singapore), under the ISR all WHO member states had legal control of epidemiological information.

In addition to the administration of international treaties and the collection of epidemiological data, since its foundation the WHO has conducted many other activities for infectious disease prevention and control, including the development of international guidelines and the coordination of global campaigns. The campaign for the eradication of smallpox (1966–1980) is often credited as one of the most important achievements of the WHO to date. Based on a combination of global surveillance, prevention measures and vaccination programmes, the campaign successfully ended the transmission of a disease that caused 300 million deaths in the twentieth century alone, largely in LMICs. Other WHO campaigns on global diseases, however, have been less successful. For example, malaria control and elimination programmes have repeatedly fallen below expectations, highlighting the many technical and institutional challenges involved in the WHO's ambitious mandate to improve health worldwide (Lee 2008).

Institutional change and global initiatives

During the 1970s, success in reducing the incidence of infectious disease in high-income countries led to complacency about the need for sustained prevention and control measures. In 1967, for example, the Surgeon General of the United States announced: 'The time has come to close the book on infectious diseases. We have basically wiped out infection in the United States' (Upshur 2008). It was also anticipated that LMICs would undergo a similar epidemiological transition, ushered in by the development of new vaccines and technologies. From the 1980s, however, the dramatic rise of malaria cases in the Global South, the emergence of AMR, the HIV/AIDS pandemic, SARS, MERS and Ebola have brought renewed emphasis on the importance of infectious disease control, while Covid-19 has clearly shown that infectious diseases can still take a huge health and economic toll on wealthy countries. Furthermore, the complexity of socio-economic challenges associated with these diseases has required novel approaches and institutional arrangements, and the active role of new actors beyond governments and established international agreements.

The case of HIV/AIDS clearly illustrates the nature of these changes. During the 1980s, the direction of early international efforts against HIV/AIDS was mainly a responsibility of the WHO, which developed a Special Programme on AIDS and a global strategy to coordinate national policies and the adoption of common guidelines. However, it soon became apparent that the global spread and complexity of this disease required the institutional support from a wider range of organizations. As a result, other specialized agencies of the United Nations became actively involved in the global campaign against HIV/AIDS, including the United Nations Development Programme (UNDP), the United Nations Population Fund (UNFPA), the United Nations Children's Emergency Fund (UNICEF), the World Bank and the Food and Agriculture Organization (FAO), providing input in their specific areas of expertise. For example, UNICEF developed several programmes on mother-to-child transmission, expanding access to treatment for pregnant and breastfeeding women living with HIV. The World Bank also become a prominent institutional actor in HIV/AIDS campaigns, partly in recognition of the link between disease burden and economic development.

In addition, a new UN programme, UNAIDS, was created to coordinate and support global action against the pandemic as further discussed in Chapter 10.

In parallel with these institutional developments, new cooperative arrangements involving the public sector along with the private sector and the civil society have emerged (see Chapter 12). Since the late 1990s, these 'global health partnerships' (also known as 'public–private partnerships') have been a dominant organizational model to support and coordinate efforts for the prevention and control of infectious diseases, involving national governments, multilateral organizations, civil society organizations (CSOs), pharmaceutical companies and charities such as the Bill and Melinda Gates Foundation; examples of global health partnerships (GHPs) include the Global Fund to fight AIDS, Tuberculosis and Malaria (the Global Fund), the World Bank's Multi-country AIDS Programme (MAP) and the GAVI Alliance on immunization. Overall, GHPs have been an effective mechanism to address complex global health issues, leading to a significant increase in aid funds and healthcare delivery, despite repeated financial crises. For example, the Global Fund has generated and managed a large budget for health, which has been used to scale up access to treatment, prevention and care services in Africa and other developing regions. In 2019, the Global Fund secured pledges of US$14.02 billion at the Sixth Replenishment Conference, the largest amount ever raised for a multilateral health organization (Global Fund 2020).

Scale-up of funds has certainly had positive effects on health outcomes – in 2018 it was estimated that health programmes supported by the Global Fund had saved 32 million lives. Yet the role and legitimacy of global health partnerships have been questioned. For example, critics have argued that the focus on 'high-profile' infectious diseases such as HIV, TB and malaria may divert resources and attention from other important public health concerns in LMICs, which are not covered by funded programmes. Furthermore, there are key issues of sustainability; funding is usually given on an ad-hoc basis to implement multi-annual programmes, but there are no mechanisms to ensure continued support in the long term.

Global surveillance

As we have seen earlier in this chapter, during the 1950s the international regime of disease surveillance was based on a set of binding rules, the International Sanitary Regulations, under which signatory states were mandated to notify the WHO of outbreaks of specific diseases and maintain adequate public health measures at key entry/exit points (e.g. seaports and airports). This approach was largely derived from the sanitary conventions of the nineteenth century and remained in place for many years. Subsequent changes included cutting back the provisions related to the annual pilgrimage to Mecca and the renaming of the ISR as International Health Regulations (IHR) in 1969 and changes in the list of notifiable diseases when smallpox was removed in 1981 after eradication (Fidler 2005).

In the late 1980s, however, it became increasingly apparent that this regulatory framework was inadequate to keep up with the pressures of globalization and associated public health challenges. First, with the compression of travelling times by air transport, the application of quarantine measures to suspected or confirmed cases was insufficient to control the transnational spread of diseases; people could contract a disease in one country and cross borders by air travel within the incubation period well before the appearance of any symptoms, as seen in the Covid-19 pandemic. Second, despite the binding nature of the IHR, WHO member states repeatedly failed to comply with the obligations of notification, often due to fears of economic losses that may result from disruptions to trade and tourism. Third, the focus on a short list of known diseases became anachronistic in the changing global health context, characterized by increasing recognition of the potential threats of novel or evolving pathogens, as captured in the concept of 'emerging infectious diseases'. Fashioned in the USA in the late 1980s, this concept has influenced global health narratives and approaches by emphasizing the links between globalizing processes and rapid microbial change and adaptation, and the resulting need for constant disease surveillance (Weir and Mykhalovskiy 2009). In the aftermath of public health crises associated with previously unknown diseases such as SARS, bovine spongiform encephalopathy (BSE), Nipah virus and avian influenza H5N1, this focus on disease surveillance became a priority on the global health agenda.

In this context, a major revision of the IHR was introduced in 2005, which substantially broadened the scope of the provisions. In the past, health authorities were mandated to report only outbreaks of certain notifiable diseases. However, the new IHRs required state parties to report 'all events which may constitute a public health emergency of international concern' (Article 6.1), based on a tool to assist decision-making (Figure 5.3). In addition, the new strategy emphasized the importance of 'early warning systems' to detect disease outbreaks or other health threats through constant monitoring of social media and international news or reports from volunteers worldwide. For example, the Global Public Health Intelligence Network (GPHIN), developed by Canada's Public Health Agency in collaboration with the WHO, is an electronic alert system, which scans online content 24/7 through specialized analysists working in nine languages and automated strategies to identify any messages that may suggest the occurrence of outbreaks. Given the unofficial nature of such sources, the WHO's Global Alert and Response Network (GOARN) is mandated to verify the reports and perform risk analysis through field missions and consultations involving national stakeholders, the WHO regional offices and other sources, and an evaluation of the potential for international spread. If the incoming report meets the required criteria for a public health event of international concern, the WHO is responsible for the dissemination of official alerts to national and international authorities, and the development of an action plan for the coordination of international response.

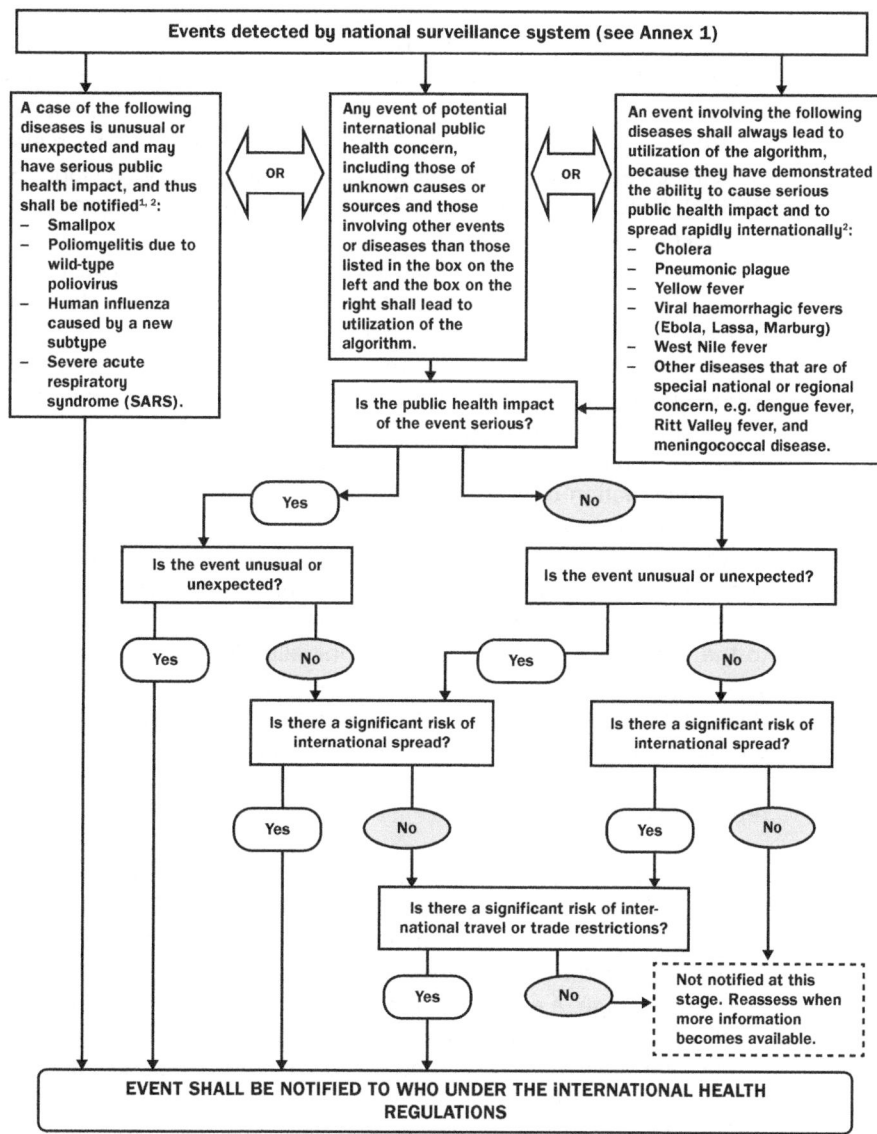

Figure 5.3: Decision instrument for the assessment and notification of events that may constitute a public health emergency of international concern in the IHR 2005

Source: Reproduced with permission from *International Health Regulations 2005*, third edition, p. 43, Copyright WHO 2016. Available at: https://globalization.who.int/publications/i/item/9789241580496 (accessed 14 April 2021).

Other systems that were established to conduct event-based global public health surveillance include MEDISYS (run by the Health Threats Unit at the Directorate General of Health and Consumer Affairs of the European Commission), Argus (hosted at the Georgetown University Medical Center and funded by the US government), Biocaster (based at the National Institute of Informatics in Tokyo), Health Map (funded by Google Inc. and located at the Harvard Medical School) and ProMED-mail (the largest publicly available system, established by the International Society for Infectious Diseases). In addition, disease surveillance networks have also been established at the regional level such as the European Surveillance System (TESSy), based at the European Centre for Disease Prevention and Control in Stockholm.

Evaluations of these initiatives have generally been positive. In 2011, for example, a report concluded that GOARN 'largely met its main aims and objectives of coordination and deployment of experts to support countries, and continues to be relevant and necessary', highlighting the large number of field missions conducted to assist outbreak investigation and response, particularly in Africa (Sondorp et al. 2011). GPHIN also gained a high international reputation for its work on disease surveillance and the detection of early signs of the 2009 swine flu pandemic in Mexico, Zika in West Africa, H5N1 in Iran, MERS and Ebola. However, recent emergencies have exposed serious shortcomings in the global response system and its ability to act quickly on information gathered by surveillance networks. During the Ebola crisis in 2014, the international response to the outbreaks in West Africa was initially slow and ineffective (Gostin and Friedman 2015). More recently, an independent evaluation of the response to Covid-19, based on hundreds of interviews and documents, concluded that the global pandemic alert system was 'not fit for purpose', with critical elements deemed 'slow, cumbersome, and indecisive'. The report concluded that:

> *Overall, the procedures and protocols attached to the operation of the International Health Regulations (2005) (IHR), including those leading up to the declaration of a public health emergency of international concern, seem to come from an earlier analogue era and need to be brought into the digital age. A system of distributed information, fed by people in local clinics and laboratories, and supported by real-time data gathering and decision-making tools, is necessary to enable reaction at the speed required – which is days, not weeks – to confront epidemic risk.* (IPPPR 2021)

The proliferation of uncoordinated surveillance networks and initiatives has been another long-standing challenge, resulting in the duplication of efforts, lack of coordination and poor integration (Calain 2007). In consideration of this, plans have been discussed to establish a 'network of networks', linking together existing local, regional, national and international networks. However, questions remain about the feasibility of such a super-surveillance system, as this would involve the solution of complex technical problems and governance challenges.

✎ Activity 5.2

Health Map is a freely available online system for real-time surveillance of emerging public health threats. It provides epidemiological intelligence by automatically aggregating disparate data sources, including official reports, online news, social media and reports from non-governmental organizations (NGOs) working in the field. Access the Health Map website (globalization.healthmap.org) and identify a recent disease outbreak in your country or another country of your choice. If you were a public health expert working in the WHO's Global Alert Response team, what steps would you take to verify the validity and threat of the outbreak information?

Feedback

Outbreak verification involves a sequence of practices, which are aimed at evaluating the validity and potential threat of the reported information. You should first evaluate the nature of the infection and the potential to spread across borders using the tool in Figure 5.3, its geographical context and the country's capacity to respond, as well as the reliability of the information source. You should then seek confirmation of details from health authorities in the countries concerned, usually through the WHO representative, and possibly also unofficial sources working in the field, such as the International Red Cross or other NGOs.

Summary

Processes of globalization have given rise to unprecedented public health challenges. Economic development and changes in food production systems have created new interactions between humans, animals and the environments that have the potential to promote the emergence of new diseases. Once diseases emerge or re-emerge, increasing mobility of people and goods within and across countries facilitates rapid and wide transmission. At the same time, the evolution of global health institutions and the emergence of new cooperative arrangements have created new opportunities to address these threats. Nonetheless, key policy challenges remain. The involvement of a diverse range of stakeholders in the global health landscape has generated substantial resources and funds to improve infectious disease control but has also resulted in the fragmentation of global health action, poor coordination and duplication of efforts. This complexity is further compounded by the emergence of new and increasingly powerful global health actors, particularly China, with governance approaches to global health and development that are different to Western donors. Most importantly, many of the benefits derived from economic globalization have disproportionately accrued to wealthy countries, leaving poor nations still vulnerable to a high burden of infectious diseases. Inequitable access to resources for the prevention, treatment and control of disease is arguably the most important challenge ahead for global health, requiring continued investments and innovative policy responses. Finally, Covid-19 has posed enormous and unprecedented global health challenges, which will certainly require stronger preparedness mechanisms and a sharper focus on health system resilience in response to infectious disease outbreaks and other challenges such as natural disasters. In an increasingly interconnected world, this can only be achieved through innovation and major reforms of the global governance architecture to ensure effective and rapid coordination between relevant stakeholders within and across countries.

References

Barnett, T. and Whiteside, A. (2002) *AIDS in the Twenty-first Century: Disease and Globalization*. Basingstoke: Palgrave Macmillan.

Briggs, A. (1961) Cholera and society in the nineteenth century, *Past and Present*, 19: 76–96.

Calain, P. (2007) From the field side of the binoculars: a different view on global public health surveillance, *Health Policy and Planning*, 22(1): 13–20.

Coker, R.J., Atun, R. and McKee, M. (2008) *Health Systems and the Challenge of Communicable Diseases: Experiences from Europe and Latin America*. Maidenhead: Open University Press.

Diamond, J. (2002) Evolution, consequences and future of plant and animal domestication, *Nature*, 418: 700-70712167878.

Elviss, N.C., Little, C.L., Hucklesby, L. et al. (2009) Microbiological study of fresh herbs from retail premises uncovers an international outbreak of salmonellosis, *International Journal of Food Microbiology*, 134(1–2): 83–88.

FAO (2017) *The Future of Food and Agriculture: Trends and Challenges*. Rome: Food and Agriculture Organization of the United Nations Rome. Available at: https://www.fao.org/3/i6583e/i6583e.pdf (accessed 4 November 2021).

Fidler, D.P. (2005) From international sanitary conventions to global health security: the new international health regulations, *Chinese Journal of International Law*, 4(2): 325–392.

Fornace, K., Liverani, M., Rushton, J. et al. (2013) Effects of land use changes and agricultural practices on the emergence and re-emergence of human viral diseases, in S. Singh (ed.) *Viral Infections and Global Change*. Hoboken, NJ: Wiley-Blackwell.

The Global Fund (2020) Results Report 2020. Available at: https://globalization.theglobalfund.org/media/10103/corporate_2020resultsreport_report_en.pdf (accessed February 2021).

Gostin, L.O. and Friedman, E.A. (2015) A retrospective and prospective analysis of the west African Ebola virus disease epidemic: robust national health systems at the foundation and an empowered WHO at the apex, *The Lancet*, 385(9980): 1902–1909.

Huber, V. (2006) The unification of the globe by disease? The international sanitary conferences on cholera, 1851–1894, *The Historical Journal*, 49: 453–476.

ICAO (2018) The world of air transport in 2018, International Civil Aviation Organization. Available at: https://globalization.icao.int/annual-report-2018/Pages/the-world-of-air-transport-in-2018.aspx (accessed 1 July 2021).

IPPPR (2021) Second report on progress. Independent Panel for Pandemic Preparedness and Response for the WHO Executive Board. January 2021. Available at: https://theindependent- panel.org/wp-content/uploads/2021/01/Independent-Panel_Second-Report-on-Progress_Final-15-Jan-2021.pdf. (accessed 12 May 2021).

Lee, K. (2008) *The World Health Organization (WHO)*. London: Routledge.

Laporta, G.Z., Ilacqua, R.C., Bergo, E.S. et al. (2021) Malaria transmission in landscapes with varying deforestation levels and timelines in the Amazon: a longitudinal spatiotemporal study, *Scientific Reports*, 11(1): 6477.

Liverani, M. and Coker, R. (2012) Protecting Europe from diseases: from the international sanitary conferences to the ECDC, *Journal of Health Politics, Policy, and Law*, 37(6): 915–934.

Liverani, M., Waage, J., Barnett, T. et al. (2013) Understanding and managing zoonotic risk in the new livestock industries, *Environmental Health Perspectives*, 121(8): 873–877.

Marcos Barba, L. van Regenmortel, H. and Ehmke, E. (2020) Shelter from the storm: the global need for universal social protection in times of Covid-19. Oxfam International. Available at: https://www.oxfam.org/en/research/shelter-storm-global-need-universal-social-protection-times-covid-19 (accessed 12 May 2021).

Morens, D.M., Folkers, G.K. and Fauci, A.S. (2009) What is a pandemic?, *The Journal of Infectious Diseases*, 200(7): 1018–1021.

O'Neill, J. (2014) *Antimicrobial Resistance: Tackling a Crisis for the Health and Wealth of Nations*. London: Wellcome Trust.

Pfeiffer, D.U., Otte, M.J., Roland-Holst, D. et al. (2011) Implications of global and regional patterns of highly pathogenic avian influenza virus H5N1 clades for risk management, *The Veterinary Journal*, 190(3): 309–316.

Piot, P. (2014) Ebola's perfect storm, *Science*, 345(6202): 1221.

Robinson, T.P., Thornton P.K., Franceschini, G. et al. (2011) *Global Livestock Production Systems*. Rome: Food and Agriculture Organization of the United Nations (FAO) and International Livestock Research Institute (ILRI).

Saker, L., Lee, K. and Cannito, B. (2007) Infectious disease in the age of globalization, in I. Kawachi and S. Wamala (eds) *Globalization and Health*. Oxford: Oxford University Press.

Sondorp, E., Ansell, C., Stevens, R.H. et al. (2011) *Independent Evaluation of the Global Outbreak and Response Network*. Geneva: World Health Organization. Available at: https://www.who.int/ihr/publications/WHO_HSE_GCR_GOARN_2011_2.pdf (accessed 4 November 2021).

Upshur, R. (2008) Ethics and infectious disease, *Bulletin of the World Health Organization*, 86(8): 654.

Vittor, A., Pan, G., Gilman, R. et al. (2009) Linking deforestation to malaria in the Amazon: characterization of the breeding habitat of the principal malaria vector, *Anopheles darlingi*, *The American Journal of Tropical Medicine and Hygiene*, 81(1): 5–12.

Weir, L. and Mykhalovskiy, E. (2009) *Global Public Health Vigilance: Creating a World on Alert*. London: Routledge.

WHO (1948) Constitution of the World Health Organization. Geneva: WHO. Available at: apps.who.int/gb/bd/PDF/bd47/EN/constitution-en.pdf (accessed 9 April 2021).

WHO (1951) *International Sanitary Regulations*. Geneva: World Health Organization.

WHO (2020) Top 10 causes of death. Available at: https://www.who.int/news-room/fact-sheets/detail/the-top-10-causes-of-death (accessed 15 March 2021).

Woods, A. (2012) Rethinking the history of modern agriculture: British pig production, c.1910–65, *20th Century British History*, 23(2): 165–191.

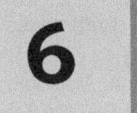

6

Globalization and non-communicable diseases

Aloisia Katsande and Benjamin Hawkins

Overview

This chapter examines the challenge posed by non-communicable diseases (NCDs) globally and the impact of globalization on our lifestyles and on the associated risk factors for NCDs. The chapter will also examine the structural causes of NCDs, how globalization influences these causes and the approaches taken to address the growing NCD burden nationally and globally.

Learning objectives

After working through this chapter, you will be able to:

- Describe the global burden of, and the main risk factors for, NCDs.
- Understand how processes of globalization affect the global burden of non-communicable disease and their associated risk factors.
- Critically assess the different approaches to understanding the nature of NCDs and the interventions to address these.

Key terms

Epidemiological transition: Changing patterns in disease, fertility, life expectancy and leading causes of death (i.e. shifts from infectious diseases to chronic diseases as the main causes of death) due to demographic, social and economic factors.

Double burden of disease: The co-existence of the burden of communicable diseases and non-communicable diseases within the same population.

Nutrition transition: Transition of diets from traditional cereal based diets to 'Western' processed diets high in sugar, salt, fats, and animal products and low in fibre and other nutrients.

The impact of NCDs globally

NCDs are non-infectious and thus, as the name suggests, non-communicable. They are generally diseases of relatively long duration and slow progression and for this reason are sometimes referred to as chronic diseases. The main types of NCDs, based on their contributions to premature mortality globally, are cardiovascular diseases (i.e. heart diseases and stroke), cancer (i.e. lung, breast, liver and colorectal cancers), chronic respiratory disease (i.e. chronic obstructive pulmonary disease [COPD] and asthma) and diabetes. However, when morbidity and disability are also taken into account, other non-communicable diseases such as mental health conditions (e.g. depression, schizophrenia, anxiety), neurological conditions (e.g. Parkinson's disease and epilepsy) and musculoskeletal conditions (e.g. arthritis and back pain) are found to be major causes of disability.

NCDs have emerged in recent decades as the leading cause of death, disease and economic burden internationally (Reubi et al. 2016). According to the World Health Organization (WHO), NCDs account for 7 of the 10 main causes of death globally and they were responsible for 74 per cent of all global deaths in 2019 (WHO 2020b). This 'epidemiological transition' from a higher burden of infectious diseases to NCDs is more apparent in high-income countries in which infectious diseases have been effectively combatted. However, a similar transition is now occurring in low- and middle-income countries (LMICs), which often experience a 'double burden' of both chronic NCDs and infectious diseases, along with enduring maternal and child health issues. Indeed, LMICs carry a disproportionate burden of NCDs, with over 85 per cent of premature deaths due to NCDs occurring in LMICs (WHO 2018b). These significant epidemiological changes are also indicated by global trends in disability-adjusted life years (DALYs), a measure of disease burden that combines mortality and healthy life 'lost' to illness. Figure 6.1 shows global changes in the five leading causes of death between 1990 and 2019.

NCDs have major adverse social, economic and health effects, and their impact stretches across the life-course. Evidence indicates that exposure to certain NCD risk factors in early life influences the development of NCDs in adulthood (Marmot and Bell 2019). For example, poor nutrition in pregnancy and childhood obesity have been associated with cardiovascular disease (CVD), diabetes and certain cancers in adulthood (Abarca-Gómez et al. 2017). WHO estimated that around 15 million people between the ages of 30 and 69 die prematurely every year from NCDs (WHO 2018b). The premature death of those in their prime productive years has a significant social and economic impact at both household level, due to loss of income and costs of healthcare, and country level, through reductions in productivity and increased costs and capacity

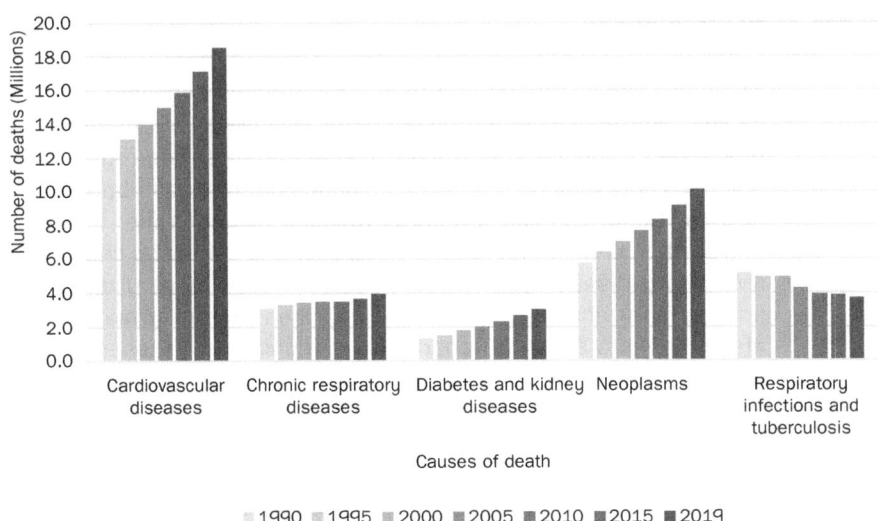

Figure 6.1: Global changes in the five leading causes of death between 1990 and 2019
Source: IHME GBD 2019 data

pressures on already strained health systems (Bloom et al. 2011b; Chaker et al. 2015).

Behavioural risk factors

There is a wide range of NCD risk factors associated with NCDs including individual behaviour and what are sometimes termed lifestyle factors such as tobacco use, alcohol consumption, unhealthy diet and physical inactivity. Furthermore, these are key drivers of intermediate risk factors – health conditions that are also implicated in the aetiology of NCDs – including overweight/obesity, elevated blood glucose, high blood pressure and high cholesterol. These risk factors are considered preventable and modifiable and are often seen to result from the choices which individuals make about their own behaviour. These risk factors are inextricably linked to processes of economic globalization (see Chapter 2), social and global environmental changes (Chapter 3 and Chapter 7) and the emergence of transnational corporations (see Chapter 11), which sell and market health-harming products in ever-increasing markets across the world as a result of trade liberalization (see Chapter 13).

However, the understanding of these risks in terms of individual behaviour or people's lifestyle choices relies on a narrow, atomized and reductionist conception of the individual separated from the societal context in which they are situated. A more sophisticated and nuanced understanding of consumption sees the individual, and the behaviours they exhibit, within what we can term the 'choice environment' in which they are located. For example, if you live in a society in which alcohol is widely marketed, healthy nutritious food is more expensive than calorie dense, nutritionally poor processed alternatives and physical activity is limited by the built environment and transportation infrastructure, then it is unsurprising that your diet, level of alcohol consumption and daily exercise – and thus your health outcomes – are constrained by this. The underlying causes of NCD are thus political, economic, socio-cultural, environmental and historical in nature. In addition, the complex set of institutions and processes through which our environments are produced and governed are increasingly complex and globalized in nature.

The public policy interventions that emerge from mainstream public health analyses – and these narrow, individualized terms in which they frame NCD risk factors – place the emphasis on individuals to manage their own exposure to such risks. For example, policy responses may focus on interventions such as public information campaigns to encourage people to exercise, eat more fruit and vegetables, drink less alcohol, quit smoking and exercise more. However, these often pay little attention to the constraints that exist for individuals to make these 'lifestyle' changes in the environments in which they live. Contextual and structural factors (e.g. the choice and affordability of food available and the marketing of these products by producers) shape and constrain the choices it is possible for individuals to make. This has implications for debates about the causes of health inequalities within countries and globally and the role of poverty and inequality as both a driver and a consequence of NCD prevalence.

Box 6.1   Behavioural risk factors for NCDs

Tobacco

Tobacco use is a key risk factor for cardiovascular diseases (CVD) and chronic respiratory conditions through direct use and second-hand smoking (WHO 2018a). Tobacco use is reducing in high-income countries (HICs), mostly due to the implementation of robust national tobacco control policies and, at the global level, the WHO Framework Convention on Tobacco Control (FCTC) (Mbulo et al. 2016). In contrast, the number of smokers has increased in many LMICs as a result of different factors including weak enforcement of control policy and the pressure of tobacco corporations (Mbulo et al. 2016). Studies have also shown that there is a strong gender divide in tobacco use (with men generally smoking at higher rates than women), although the extent of this varies between regions (Mackay 2012).

Alcohol

Excessive alcohol use has been linked to multiple cancers (e.g. of the oral cavity, pharynx, larynx, oesophagus, liver and breast), CVD, liver diseases, maternal and perinatal conditions and depression (WHO 2018a). In 2016, over 3 million deaths and 136.6 million DALYs globally were attributed to alcohol (WHO 2018a). Alcohol use patterns differ between regions, countries, socio-economic groups and genders. While those of higher socio-economic status (SES) are more likely to drink alcohol, the burden of harm from alcohol use is concentrated in lower SES (WHO 2018a; Sadler et al. 2017). This 'alcohol harm paradox' has been observed between countries, with LMICs experiencing a higher burden of disease and deaths attributable to alcohol (measured by DALYs and deaths), despite lower consumption rates compared to HICs (WHO 2018a). According to WHO, Africa is the region with the highest burden of alcohol-attributed disease, while Europe has the highest alcohol consumption but lower levels of harm (WHO 2018a). This suggests that NCDs are the result of a complex inter-play of different risk factors of which alcohol is only one. Studies have found also that a combination of high levels of alcohol consumption and poverty is a key driver of mortality and morbidity, at least in high-income settings (Katikireddi et al. 2017).

Diet
Unhealthy diets contribute to hypertension, high cholesterol and obesity, which are important risk factors for CVDs, diabetes, stroke and certain cancers. In 2019, unhealthy diets were responsible for over 7 million deaths among adults aged 25 and older and 188 million DALYs worldwide (IHME 2019b). Notably, levels of obesity have significantly increased over the past few decades. Moreover, the lack of adequate nutrients and micronutrients in diets is a further risk factor, especially in LMIC settings. It is important to note that countries, cities, households and even individuals may experience a double burden of overweight and malnutrition. Processes of globalization have led to shifts away from traditional cereal based diets to 'Western' diets and processed foods, particularly in LMICs (Popkin et al. 2012). These diets have become increasingly common in LMICs resulting in increases in diet related ill-health (Popkin et al. 2012) (Chapters 2 and 3).

Physical inactivity
Physical inactivity is a key risk factor for NCDs such as CVDs, diabetes and cancer and is estimated to cause between 4 and 5 million preventable deaths every year. According to WHO (2020a), 1 in 4 adults globally do not meet WHO's recommended levels of exercise with these figures even higher for school-aged children (Guthold et al. 2020). As with the nutritional transition discussed above, these trends are associated with wider structural and socio-economic changes globally (Holtermann et al. 2018).

🖉 **Activity 6.1**

Go to the Institute of Health Metrics and Evaluation (IHME) at http://
www.healthdata.org/results/country-profiles, and select a high-income,
a middle-income and a low-middle income country (one of which could be
your country). Compare and contrast the main causes of death and disability between these countries. What is the contribution of NCDs to the
overall burden of disease in these countries? Which specific diseases
account for this? How does this vary between the countries? What factors might explain this?

Feedback

You may have noted some of the following:

- There might be a double burden of infectious diseases and NCDs in
  LMICs.
- Infectious diseases are the main cause of death in some LMICs.
- NCDs are the main causes of death and disability in some HICs.
- Changes in the main causes of death between 1990 and 2019, as
  NCDs become increasingly prevalent in LMICs and there is a reduc-
  tion in infectious diseases (epidemiological transition).
- Other NCDs such as neurological, mental health, headache disorders
  are also significant causes of death and disability.
- HICs tend to have an ageing population compared to LMICs (though
  projections show LMICs having increasingly ageing populations).
- The leading risk factors for NCDs vary between the different income
  levels.

Globalization and structural determinants of NCDs

The conditions in which people are born, live and work have an impact on
their health (including NCDs), and processes of globalization have shaped
these conditions in various and significant ways. Increases in the movement of goods across borders, produced by globally active transnational
corporations, has led to greater availability and promotion of health-harming
products. The movement of goods across the globe, allied to extensive
industrialization in more areas of the globe have implications for climate
change and the environmental determinants of health. At the same time,
the increasing ease with which information can cross borders – what was
termed in Chapter 1 the cognitive dimension of globalization – and the
proliferation of new technologies, have led to cultural and lifestyle changes
implicated in the rise of NCDs.

Economic factors influencing the global increase of NCDs

Chapter 2 discussed the links of globalization and economic trends, including poverty. The relationship between poverty and NCDs is not unidirectional. Poverty is not just a risk factor for NCDs; the latter also have a significant causal impact on poverty (WHO 2011). Poverty shapes individual or household access to resources and amenities such as food, housing, clean energy, good employment and working conditions. For example, poor access to nutritional food or clean energy sources for cooking and heating might result in poor dietary intake and increased exposure to air pollution, increasing the likelihood of developing NCDs. Employment, poor education, housing and undernutrition are all factors that are associated with poverty and increased exposure to NCD risks (Marmot and Bell 2019). As noted, NCD prevalence can further exacerbate poverty, creating a self-reinforcing cycle of poverty and disease within families and communities.

Commercial factors influencing the global increase of NCDs

Risk factors for NCDs are strongly associated with the activities of businesses, particularly transnational corporations (TNCs), which sell and market health-harming products such as tobacco, alcohol and processed food. These companies have been identified as 'commercial determinants of health' (Kickbusch et al. 2016). Processes of trade liberalization (see Chapter 13) have led to the entry of new products and new commercial actors into markets across the world. As political scrutiny and regulatory oversight of their products and activities has increased in their 'home' markets (in many cases high-income settings such as Europe, North America and Japan), both the global tobacco and alcohol industries, for example, have increasingly focused their market strategies on populous and increasingly affluent LMICs (Hawkins et al. 2018).

Transnational companies bring with them sophisticated marketing strategies and brands and drive sales of their products in ways that can have significant population level effects on consumption patterns. In addition, transnational corporations play a key role in shaping national policies as they have the political and economic power to influence the political environment to suit their interests (see Chapter 11). This is particularly evident in LMICs where governance capacity may be limited (Glasgow and Schrecker 2015; Lencucha and Thow 2019).

The proliferation of trade and investment agreements in recent years has increased the flow of goods, processes and technologies, reshaping local food systems (see Chapter 13). Similarly, agricultural policies, driven by globalization, including those that emphasize the production of cash crops such as tobacco for export and the growing dependence on imports of staple foods have led to changes in lifestyles and consumption patterns, with implications for NCDs in both HICs and LMICs.

Socio-cultural factors

As Chapter 3 discussed, not only has trade increased access to these products, development in communications technology (e.g. television, smartphones, the internet and social media) and the flow of information globally has played a key role in shifting consumption patterns away from traditional diets (Wilson and McLennan 2019). Alcohol and tobacco companies have marketed their products as luxury brands despite their deleterious effect on health (Hawkins et al. 2018). Furthermore, their marketing activities have played a key role in introducing smoking and drinking as cultural practices in environments in which they were previously absent and have targeted particular sub-populations such as women and young people who may have previously been less likely to use their products.

Air pollution and other environmental factors

There is a wide consensus that air pollution is a major risk factor for NCDs. In the past two decades, levels of air pollution have declined in HICs, but they have risen sharply in LMICs over the same period, threatening public health and economic development (Landrigan et al. 2018). It is currently estimated that more than 90 per cent of people breathe air containing high levels of pollutants that exceed the WHO global air quality guidelines, with the highest exposures in LMICs (Shaddick et al. 2020). In addition to outdoor pollution, the use of open fires, solid fuels (such as coal, wood and crop wastes) and paraffin (or kerosene) for cooking or heating is a significant contributor to household air pollution, particularly in LMICs, and disproportionately affects women and children. In 2019, air pollution – both outdoor and indoor – was the single most important environmental cause of disease and premature death worldwide, contributing to 213 million DALYs and 6.67 million deaths (IHME 2019a). Our physical environment is also a key factor structuring NCD risk.

Chapter 3 discussed social change including urbanization and shifts in work and livelihoods. Evidence shows that in some settings a built environment (i.e. man-made infrastructures such as cities/towns, roads, neighbourhoods and parks) that is designed to encourage health promoting behaviours such as walking and other physical activities has a protective effect on some NCD risk factors, such as obesity (Michael et al. 2014). Processes of globalization-led urbanization have had significant effects on living and working conditions, access to open spaces, population density and housing quality with consequences for NCD prevalence. As will be discussed in Chapter 7, global environmental change represents a range of risks to human health, including NCDs. Evidence has shown that climate change can impact NCD risk through changes in food production, heat exposure and air pollution, resulting in obesity/overweight, undernutrition,

COPD, asthma and CVDs (Frumkin and Haines 2019). Land use changes and agricultural practices can also affect access to healthy foods and exposure to chemicals.

✎ Activity 6.2

Addressing the growing NCD burden requires joined up governmental responses that go beyond what are traditionally considered to be the focus of 'health policy'. What other policy areas do you think are important for addressing the increase in NCDs and why? How are these policy areas affected by globalization? Make some notes based on what you have read so far here and elsewhere. Draw on relevant personal experience also.

Feedback

You might have noted that while health policies, i.e. access to healthcare and preventative services, are important, they are not the only important policies to address in order to tackle NCDs and risk factors. Some of the important policies you might have come up with include multi-sectoral public policies related to the structural determinants of health such as:

- Education *(i.e. levels of educational inequalities and attainment are closely associated with higher incidences of certain NCDs).*
- Housing *(i.e. quality and characteristics of housing and neighbourhoods can influence NCDs. For example, damp housing can exacerbate respiratory conditions).*
- Agricultural policies *(can influence the supply chain in ways that increase the availability of unhealthy products).*
- Trade *(some trade policies can exacerbate inequalities and the promotion and availability of products that are detrimental to health).*
- Fiscal policies *(can help correct market failures and can provide incentives to reduce consumption of unhealthy products, for example, taxation of tobacco products and alcohol).*
- Environmental policies *(e.g. can determine levels of exposure to pollution and other environmental factors that influence NCDs).*
- Workplace and employment policies *(these can influence working conditions such as working with pesticides, asbestos, etc. and employment opportunities).*
- Urban planning and design *(influence the design of neighbourhoods, green spaces [e.g. parks] and road networks for example, which influence physical activity and access to healthy foods).*

Many of these policy areas will be affected directly or indirectly by processes of globalization. Trade, including international agreements, increases cross-border movement of goods and services (see Chapter 13), which also impacts on levels of pollution and environmental degradation (see Chapter 7). These agreements may also influence working conditions and labour rights and may lead to shifts in population distribution to towns and cities where this leads to industrialization or changes in the structure of the economy. This in turn affects housing and the wider environment in which people live. Finally, all these processes may affect government revenue and public funds available to pay for education, health and other social policies that affect health (see Chapter 2).

Behavioural vs structural approaches to address NCDs

The question of how to address NCD risk factors can be approached in different ways and at a different levels. Here we identify three approaches that can be referred to as the *individual*, *structural* and *system* levels. As noted above, individual approaches focus on issues such as diet, physical activity and tobacco and alcohol use as the key determinants of NCDs, while emphasizing the role of genetics in determining NCD prevalence. This perspective emphasizes the role of individual choice and responsibility, and leads to the promotion of interventions – such as product labelling and public information campaigns – which aim to facilitate people to make healthier lifestyle choices.

Structural approaches, by contrast, focus on the contextual risk factors as opposed to individual behaviours. They see NCDs as societal rather than individual phenomena which require 'upstream,' population level interventions to address them. This includes the production of healthy spatial environments, living and working conditions as well as the population level regulation of health-harming commodities and practices such as tobacco, alcohol and food marketing and environmental degradation. While we may accept that individual actions play a role in health outcomes, structural approaches recognize that the choices we make are constrained by the context in which we make them. It is harder to take regular exercise if there are not open spaces available to use or paths to cycle on and it is harder to choose a healthy diet where processed foods are both cheap and heavily marketed. No individual acting alone can control the quality of air they breathe.

Finally, the systemic approach argues that even structural changes to address the upstream determinants of NCDs are inadequate and call for a radical re-orientation of society and the global economy. This involves a fundamental rejection of neo-liberal models of production and social organization and is associated with certain aspects of the environment movement and anti-capitalist movements.

Individual approaches remain the dominant policy model for addressing NCD risk factors globally. However, there is little evidence that such proximal or 'downstream' interventions on their own really work to reduce things like alcohol related harm and unhealthy diets (Babor 2010; Afshin et al. 2017). Structural approaches are identified as more effective and cost effective ways of reducing harms and promoting public health, as seen in the WHO 'Best Buys' (Bloom et al. 2011a; WHO 2017). The language of individual lifestyle 'choices' as the main causes of NCDs shifts attention from the structural factors that shape health and disease, including the role of the transnational corporations in increasing NCD mortality and morbidity globally (Glasgow and Schrecker 2015). If we accept that contextual factors such as poverty at the very least limit individual choice and individual framing of NCDs runs the danger of blaming the victims of structural factors beyond their control for the poor health they suffer. Moreover, the potential stigma associated with this framing may further exacerbate poor health (e.g. mental health) and health inequalities. While for some population subgroups (particularly those with established disease) individual-level lifestyle interventions may sometimes be beneficial, at a population level such interventions are not enough (Allen et al. 2018; Yang et al. 2018).

Structural approaches are widely opposed by private sector actors – such as the alcohol and food industries – whose business models and sales may be affected by stricter regulation and reduced consumption (see Chapter 11). Citizens may also be reluctant to support policies that they perceive as restricting their choice by limiting the availability of certain products, increasing their price or restricting their use. Politicians may be reluctant to support structural changes that might threaten certain powerful industries, for example the food, alcohol, tobacco and automotive industries, and/or be unpopular among their electorates. At the very least they need to expend a significant amount of political capital to adopt them, which may serve as a deterrent to taking such approaches. Effective interventions to address NCDs are challenging and require careful planning, appropriate infrastructure, political buy-in and multi-sectoral working across policy domains.

Global responses to NCDs

Recent decades have seen an increasing recognition of NCDs as global health issues and an increasing attempt to develop coordinated policy responses at the global level. These include the WHO Framework Convention for Tobacco Control (FCTC), the Political Declaration on the Prevention and Control of NCDs, and WHO's 25×25 strategy. These are global agreements that provide a framework for action at the national level.

WHO Framework Convention for Tobacco Control (WHO FCTC)

The WHO FCTC is the first international treaty to be negotiated under the auspices of WHO (WHO 2003). The treaty was developed as a global strategy to tackle the tobacco epidemic that was fuelled by globalization factors such as trade liberalization, transnational tobacco advertising, marketing and promotion. It came into force in February 2005 and aims to reduce the demand and supply of tobacco products in order to reduce harmful tobacco consumption and counteract the tobacco industry's activities such as lobbying, advertising and promotion activities (WHO 2003). FCTC key measures include monitoring tobacco use; implementation of smoke-free laws; tobacco cessation interventions; health warnings; banning tobacco advertising, promotion and sponsorship; and tobacco tax increases. In addition, Article 5.3 requires signatory governments to act to ward against the undue influence of the tobacco industry over policy.

UN Political Declaration on the Prevention and Control of NCDs

Heads of state met in 2011 at the United Nations for a High Level Meeting (HLM) on NCDs, which resulted in a political declaration to address the prevention and control of NCDs worldwide, with a particular focus on addressing the four key risk factors for NCD (tobacco use, unhealthy diet, physical inactivity and harmful use of alcohol) (United Nations General Assembly 2012). This political declaration was a key milestone as it was only the second time in history such a meeting had been held to address a health concern (the first one being on HIV/AIDS in 2001). It recognized the need to shift how NCDs and development were viewed and conceptualized NCDs as a developmental issue and a threat to economies, health, sustainable development and other social challenges. Subsequent HLMs on NCDs were held in 2014 and 2018. While these were significant events, the progress in NCDs has been considered slow and inadequate, particularly in the deployment of resources and policies to address NCDs at global and regional levels (Suzuki et al. 2021).

WHO 25×25 strategy

The WHO framework set out NCD targets to be met by all member states by 2025. The 25×25 strategy sets out nine global voluntary targets with the overarching aim to reduce premature death from the four major NCDs by 25 per cent by 2025. It mainly focuses on reducing mortality from four main NCDs (cardiovascular disease, diabetes, cancer and chronic respiratory disease) by targeting the four risk factors, i.e. physical inactivity, tobacco use, harmful alcohol use and unhealthy diets. However, one of the key criticisms of this approach is that its focus on mortality overlooks the high burden of morbidity due to NCDs, and it does not consider other key NCDs such as mental illness and musculoskeletal conditions such as arthritis and lower back pain.

These global governance measures have had some degree of success in triggering policy reforms nationally and globally and remain a key part of the policy architecture in tackling the increase in NCDs. For example, the FCTC has served as a strong normative force for tobacco control advocates to hold signatory governments to account for the international commitments they have made in signing and ratifying this agreement. The absence of such a global framework has similarly undermined efforts to advocate for more robust policy regime approaches to industry actors in areas such as alcohol and food policy. This has led some public health actors to argue for the creation of a Framework Convention on Global Health, which would address NCD risk factors beyond tobacco (Friedman et al. 2013).

When designing public health interventions to tackle the NCD burden in a globalized world, there is need to be cognizant of the historical legacies that have led to the creation of power imbalances and vulnerabilities. Public health interventions are often ahistorical, addressing current issues and problems without due acknowledgement of the historical structures that shaped these (Wilson and McLennan 2019). Similarly, one-size-fits-all interventions will not be appropriate and there is need to examine how the local context (i.e. social, economic, political and historical context) interplays with the global in shaping patterns of diseases and finding solutions that are appropriate to the local context. It is too simplistic to assume that determinants of health are homogeneous and that national priorities are the same (Eshetu and Woldesenbet 2011). Countries have different levels of economic development, public service provision (i.e. healthcare, sanitation, governance systems) and other social challenges that influence action or inaction in meeting the global NCD targets. Slow progress on NCDs has been blamed on inadequate funding, weak health systems, the poor framing of NCDs as a policy challenge and industry opposition (Yang et al. 2020). The danger remains that some global NCD policies that focus on individual risk factors fail to address the conditions that underlie people's exposure to risks and disease, further exacerbating inequalities and ill health (Prince 2014).

Furthermore, the power imbalances that exist in global health governance have implications for the influence of stakeholders. For example, some high-income countries and industries oppose stricter regulatory policy options for addressing health-harming products such as alcohol (Suzuki et al. 2021). This imbalance is also evident in NCD evidence generation. Evidence has been used to generate recommendations for NCD policies and interventions (Reubi et al. 2016); however, despite the disproportionate distribution of the burden of NCDs in LMICs, much of the NCD research is from HICs, and LMICs remain underrepresented (Heneghan et al. 2013), and this could potentially impact on how they progress in relation to implementing global NCD policies.

Some have pointed to limited funds, weak health systems, poor framing and articulation of NCDs to the public, and the sheer complexity of an NCD-specific challenge as obstacles to progress (Yang et al. 2020). What has received less attention is whether evidence-based interventions within the scientific literature and recommended by global institutions are acceptable to national governments and can be effectively implemented by member states.

Activity 6.3

How effective would a framework convention on global health (FCGH) be in addressing NCDs globally? What are the potential barriers to creating and implementing such an agreement? What alternatives exist to implementing an FCGH? What are the advantages and disadvantages of these?

Feedback

The experience of the FCTC suggests that the consequences of these agreements can be important, but should not be overstated. They create a global policy consensus that health advocates, nationally and globally, can use to lobby governments for effective policy changes by holding them to the internationally agreed 'best practice' to which they have committed and using comparisons with other states that are adopting the agreed measures. However, implementation of the FCTC has been piecemeal and limited and attempts to create further protocols to flesh out the convention have proven hard to agree and ratify (see Fooks et al. 2017). This is in a single policy area in which the harms of the product and the industry are widely accepted. Trying to replicate this across areas is likely to mean that agreement on a text and adoption in member states and international organizations will be even harder to obtain. And this is before the issues of effective implementation, noted above. Such an agreement is likely to face huge opposition from multiple sectors including corporations in the food, alcohol and polluting industries in the same way that 'big tobacco' opposed the FCTC. This has led some to call for individual sectoral conventions (e.g. on alcohol and food). However, these run the danger of or playing off health issues against each other when advocates in each area have shared interests and concerns for health and the effective treatment of NCDs requires a joined up and multi-sectoral approach.

Summary

This chapter examined the global burden of NCDs and the different ways of understanding the drivers of the global NCD crisis and the appropriate policy response to this. The rise in NCDs is the consequence of various structural risk factors that have been influenced and exacerbated by processes of globalization. These risk factors, and the resulting NCD burden, are not evenly distributed either between or within states globally with some (often the poorest) countries and populations disproportionately at risk from, and affected by, NCDs. The chapter argued that individualized framings of NCDs and targeted policy responses that follow from this are inadequate in reducing NCD prevalence globally. Instead, structural factors need to be addressed to reverse current trends. The 'upstream' nature of many determinants of NCD – such as environmental degradation, food systems and unhealthy commodity marketing – means that effective policy interventions to address these must be focused at the population level to address structural risk factors, including action in sectors outside the remit of what is traditionally considered health policy.

References

Abarca-Gómez, L., Abdeen, Z.A., Hamid, Z.A. et al. (2017) Worldwide trends in body-mass index, underweight, overweight, and obesity from 1975 to 2016: a pooled analysis of 2416 population-based measurement studies in 128.9 million children, adolescents, and adults, *The Lancet*, 390: 2627–2642.

Afshin, A., Micha, R., Webb, M. et al. (2017) Effectiveness of dietary policies to reduce noncommunicable diseases, in D. Prabhakaran, S. Anand, T.A. Gaziano et al. (eds) *Cardiovascular, Respiratory, and Related Disorders*. Washington, DC: The International Bank for Reconstruction and Development/The World Bank.

Allen, L.N., Pullar, J., Wickramasinghe, K.K. et al. (2018) Evaluation of research on interventions aligned to WHO 'Best Buys' for NCDs in low-income and lower-middle-income countries: a systematic review from 1990 to 2015, *BMJ Global Health*, 3: e000535.

Babor, T. (2010) *Alcohol: No Ordinary Commodity: Research and Public Policy*. Oxford: Oxford University Press.

Bloom, D.E., Cafiero, E.T., Jané-Llopis, E. et al. (2011b) *The Global Economic Burden of Noncommunicable Diseases*. Geneva: World Economic Forum.

Bloom, D., Chisholm, D., Jane Llopis, E. et al. (2011a) *From Burden to 'Best Buys': Reducing the Economic Impact of Non-Communicable Disease in Low and Middle-Income Countries*. Geneva: World Economic Forum.

Chaker, L., Falla, A., van der Lee, S.J. et al. (2015) The global impact of non-communicable diseases on macro-economic productivity: a systematic review, *European Journal of Epidemiology*, 30: 357–395.

Eshetu, E.B. and Woldesenbet, S.A. (2011) Are there particular social determinants of health for the world's poorest countries?, *African Health Sciences*, 11: 108–115.

Fooks, G.J., Smith, J., Lee, K. et al. (2017) Controlling corporate influence in health policy making? An assessment of the implementation of article 5.3 of the World Health Organization framework convention on tobacco control, *Global Health*, 13: 12.

Friedman, E., Gostin, L. and Buse, K. (2013) Advancing the right to health through global organizations: the potential role of a Framework Convention on Global Health, *Health and Human Rights*, 6: 71–86.

Frumkin, H. and Haines, A. (2019) Global environmental change and noncommunicable disease risks, *Annual Review of Public Health*, 40: 261–282.

Glasgow, S. and Schrecker, T. (2015) The double burden of neoliberalism? Noncommunicable disease policies and the global political economy of risk, *Health & Place*, 34: 279–286.

Guthold, R., Stevens, G.A., Riley, L.M. et al. (2020) Global trends in insufficient physical activity among adolescents: a pooled analysis of 298 population-based surveys with 1.6 million participants, *The Lancet Child & Adolescent Health*, 4: 23–35.

Hawkins, B., Holden, C., Eckhardt, J. et al. (2018) Reassessing policy paradigms: a comparison of the global tobacco and alcohol industries, *Global Public Health*, 13: 1–19.

Heneghan, C., Blacklock, C., Perera, R. et al. (2013). Evidence for non-communicable diseases: analysis of Cochrane reviews and randomised trials by World Bank classification, *BMJ Open*, 3(7): e003298.

Holtermann, A., Krause, N., van der Beek, A.J. et al. (2018) The physical activity paradox: six reasons why occupational physical activity (OPA) does not confer the cardiovascular health benefits that leisure time physical activity does, *British Journal of Sports Medicine*, 52: 149.

IHME (2019a) GBD 2019 cause and risk summaries: air pollution – level 2 risk. 2021. Available at: http://www.healthdata.org/results/gbd_summaries/2019/air-pollution-level-2-risk (accessed 28 March 2021).

IHME (2019b) GBD 2019 cause and risk summaries: dietary risks – level 2 risk. 2020. Available at: http://www.healthdata.org/results/gbd_summaries/2019/dietary-risks-level-2-risk (accessed 18 February 2021).

Katikireddi, S.V., Whitley, E., Lewsey, J. et al. (2017) Socioeconomic status as an effect modifier of alcohol consumption and harm: analysis of linked cohort data, *The Lancet Public Health*, 2: e267–e276.

Kickbusch, I., Allen, L. and Franz, C. (2016) The commercial determinants of health, *The Lancet Global Health*, 4: e895–e896.

Landrigan, P.J., Fuller, R., Acosta, N.J.R. et al. (2018) The Lancet Commission on pollution and health, *The Lancet*, 391: 462–512.

Lencucha, R. and Thow, A.M. (2019) How neoliberalism is shaping the supply of unhealthy commodities and what this means for NCD prevention, *International Journal of Health Policy and Management*, 8: 514–520.

Mackay, J. (2012) The global epidemiology of tobacco and related chronic diseases, *Public Health*, 126: 199–201.

Marmot, M. and Bell, R. (2019) Social determinants and non-communicable diseases: time for integrated action, *BMJ*, 364: l251.

Mbulo, L., Ogbonna, N., Olarewaju, I. et al. (2016) Preventing tobacco epidemic in LMICs with low tobacco use – using Nigeria GATS to review WHO MPOWER tobacco indicators and prevention strategies, *Preventive Medicine*, 91: S9–S15.

Michael, Y.L., Nagel, C.L., Gold, R. et al. (2014) Does change in the neighborhood environment prevent obesity in older women?, *Social Science & Medicine*, 102: 129–137.

Popkin, B.M., Adair, L.S. and Ng, S.W. (2012) Global nutrition transition and the pandemic of obesity in developing countries, *Nutrition Reviews*, 70: 3–21.

Prince, R. (2014) Navigating 'global health' in an East African city, in R.J. Prince and R. Marsland (eds) *Making and Unmaking Public Health in Africa: Ethnographic and Historical Perspectives*. Athens: Ohio University Press.

Reubi, D., Herrick, C. and Brown, T. (2016) The politics of non-communicable diseases in the Global South, *Health & Place*, 39: 179–187.

Sadler, S., Angus, C., Gavens, L. et al. (2017) Understanding the alcohol harm paradox: an analysis of sex- and condition-specific hospital admissions by socio-economic group for alcohol-associated conditions in England, *Addiction*, 112: 808–817.

Shaddick, G., Thomas, M.L., Mudu, P. et al. (2020) Half the world's population are exposed to increasing air pollution, *Climate and Atmospheric Science*, 3: 23.

Suzuki, M., Webb, D. and Small, R. (2021) Competing frames in global health governance: an analysis of stakeholder influence on the political declaration on non-communicable diseases, *International Journal of Health Policy and Management*. Available at: https://doi.org/10.34172/IJHPM.2020.257.

United Nations General Assembly (2012) Resolution adopted by the General Assembly: 66/2: Political Declaration of the High-level Meeting of the General Assembly on the Prevention and Control of Non-communicable Diseases. Adopted 19 September 2011. Available at: https://www.who.int/nmh/events/un_ncd_summit2011/political_declaration_en.pdf (accessed 9 April 2021).

WHO (2003) Framework convention on tobacco control. Available at: https://apps.who.int/iris/bitstream/handle/10665/42811/9241591013.pdf (accessed 5 November 2021).

WHO (2011) Global status report on noncommunicable diseases 2010. Available at: https://www.who.int/nmh/publications/ncd_report2010/en/ (accessed 8 April 2021).

WHO (2017) *Tackling NCDs: 'Best Buys' and Other Recommended Interventions for the Prevention and Control of Noncommunicable Diseases*. Geneva: World Health Organization.

WHO (2018a) *Global Status Report on Alcohol and Health 2018*. Geneva: World Health Organization.

WHO (2018b) Non-communicable diseases: key facts. 2019. Available at: https://www.who.int/news-room/fact-sheets/detail/noncommunicable-diseases (accessed 20 March 2019).

WHO (2020a) Physical activity – key facts. 2021. Available at: https://www.who.int/news-room/fact-sheets/detail/physical-activity (accessed 26 November 2020).

WHO (2020b) Top 10 causes of death. Available at: https://www.who.int/news-room/fact-sheets/detail/the-top-10-causes-of-death (accessed 15 March 2021).

Wilson, M. and McLennan, A. (2019) A comparative ethnography of nutrition interventions: structural violence and the industrialisation of agrifood systems in the Caribbean and the Pacific, *Social Science & Medicine*, 228: 172–180.

Yang, J.S., Mamudu, H.M. and John, R. (2018) Incorporating a structural approach to reducing the burden of non-communicable diseases, *Globalization and Health*, 14: 66.

Yang, J.S., Mamudu, H.M. and Mackey, T.K. (2020) Governing noncommunicable diseases through political rationality and technologies of government: a discourse analysis, *International Journal of Environmental Research and Public Health*, 17(12): 4413.

Globalization, environmental change and human health

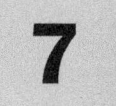

Carolyn Stephens

Overview

In this chapter, you will explore the impacts of globalization on global environmental change (GEC) and consider its related effects on human health. The chapter will begin by examining GEC, how it relates to globalization (a mix of economic, social, cultural, technological, physical and other changes), and then look at the types of health impacts GEC might have, both now and in the future. The chapter will review a range of global policy approaches to address global environmental changes and health.

Learning objectives

After working through this chapter, you will be able to:

- Distinguish global environmental change (GEC) from more traditional environmental hazards.
- Understand how GEC relates to globalization.
- Recognize the ways in which GEC, directly and indirectly, affects human health.
- Understand some of the limitations of the conceptualization of GEC and its links to human health.
- Understand a range of global policies aimed at tackling GEC.

Key terms

Biodiversity: The abundance and distributions of and interactions between genotypes, species, communities, ecosystems and biomes.

Carrying capacity: The size of population that can be indefinitely supported by the natural resource base of the specified geographic area.

Climate change: Long-term change (over decades, centuries or millennia) in average meteorological conditions (such as temperature and rainfall).

Ecosystem: The complex of a community of organisms and its environment functioning as an ecological unit.

Extreme weather events: Extreme transient weather conditions, which differ from longer-term conditions that define a prevailing *climate*.

Global environmental change: Large-scale, mostly human-induced, changes in the Earth's natural environment in recent decades as a reflection of unprecedented impacts on the biosphere.

Anthropocene era: the idea of an epoch dating from signs of significant human impact on Earth's geological and ecological systems, including anthropogenic climate change.

Understanding global environmental change

Humans, and all other species, depend upon the world's complex geophysical and ecological systems to sustain their health and survival. Humans have understood for centuries that this natural environment provides air, food and water, and a range of life-supporting environmental 'goods' (e.g. clothing materials, shelter and energy). More recently, it has become clear that 'ecosystem services' from the global environment are also critical for human survival (e.g. constancy of local climate, pollination of food plants, and the uptake of carbon dioxide and production of oxygen via plant photosynthesis) (WHO 2021). The historical record suggests that failure to maintain the natural environmental resource base has been a recurring cause of societal instability, decline and collapse (McMichael 1993). Globalization, as we saw in Chapters 1, 2 and 3, is associated with increased trade, consumption and movement of people – all of which have impacts on global environmental conditions.

Global environmental change (GEC)

During the past two centuries, human impact on the environment has increased dramatically. Human populations expanded approximately eight-fold and the material-intensity and energy-intensity of economic activity increased exponentially (Venter et al. 2016; UNDP 2020). As we discussed in Chapter 3, the world has gone through major urbanization, with impacts on health and on the global environment. The world's population, currently 7 billion, is expected to reach almost 10 billion by 2050 (UNDESA 2019). The total human 'carrying capacity' of Earth is neither fixed nor certain and depends on future patterns of consumption and waste generation (UNEP-GEAS 2012; UNDP 2020). Meanwhile, moderate and severe global food insecurity rose between 2015 and 2019 and affects an estimated 26 per cent of the world's population (UNDP 2020). Today, we face unfamiliar problems posed by global environmental change.

Box 7.1 shows some of the most important global environmental changes:

Box 7.1 Some key global environmental changes

- Global climate change, occurring in response to the excessive emission of greenhouse gases into the lower atmosphere, especially the release of carbon dioxide from fossil fuel combustion.
- Human-induced changes to the middle atmosphere (stratosphere) resulting in depletion of (ultraviolet-shielding) stratospheric ozone.
- Urbanization:
  - Land-use changes.
  - Industrialization and pollution of water and air resources.
  - Pressure on regional ecosystems.
- Massive waste generation – and displacement of waste across land and marine landscapes.
- Biodiversity change:
  - Massive loss/extinction of species.
  - Significant redistribution of species (including invasion).
- Changes to agriculture/food-producing/water supporting ecosystems:
  - Land cover, loss of soil fertility.
  - Major coastal and ocean ecosystem level destruction (including fisheries).
- Changes to the hydrological cycle; depletion of freshwater supplies including major underground aquifers; desertification, wetland and land degradation.

Human alteration of Earth and its 'operating system', including on a global scale (historically unprecedented), is now substantial and growing. It is calculated that over 75 per cent of the planet's land area is experiencing measurable human pressures (Venter et al. 2016). Estimates now put extinction of all species, other than humans, as part of an ongoing and very rapid human-driven extinction crisis – 'The Sixth Extinction' (UNDP 2020). The age of human domination and its disruptions of planetary resources and functioning has now been named the *Anthropocene era* – to follow the 11,000-year climatically stable and warmer Holocene that emerged after the last cold glacial period ('ice age') (Lewis and Maslin 2015).

Relationship of global environmental changes to globalization

As Chapter 1 explains, globalization describes a set of global processes that are intensifying the interconnected nature of human interaction across economic, political, cultural and environmental spheres. To date, almost all evidence suggests that there is a close *negative* connection between globalization and most large-scale global environmental changes (UNDP 2020). For example, there is now evidence that trade liberalization, discussed in Chapter 13, has a strong influence on deforestation, particularly through agricultural land expansion in Africa, Asia and Latin America, suggesting that 'trade liberalization not only increases net deforestation but may also shift deforestation into ecologically sensitive locations' (Abman and Lundberg 2020). As Chapter 3 shows, aspects of urbanization and industrialization are linked to increased consumption patterns. As consumption increases, particularly of energy-intensive products such as cars, heating and cooling mechanisms, and other products of urban living, the emission of greenhouse gases increases. Perhaps in response to the evidence of these negative impacts, the world's peoples also show an increasing concern to live in a 'sustainable' future world, which will presumably be a globalized world – where we work together to protect the planet and its resources (UNDP and University of Oxford 2021).

Conceptualizing the relationship of GEC to human health and well-being

In 2000 the United Nations published the Millennium Ecosystem Assessment and put forward a new conceptual model for understanding the relationship of human health and the ecosystem. This was the idea of 'Ecosystem Services for Health'. It moved our conceptual understanding of environmental health risks fundamentally from the local to the global. Figure 7.1 shows this. Conceptually, this model organizes all elements on the planet into a set of ecosystem services for human well-being – structured into supporting, provisioning, regulating and cultural services. This then links to aspects of our well-being, including security, basic material services, health and good social relations.

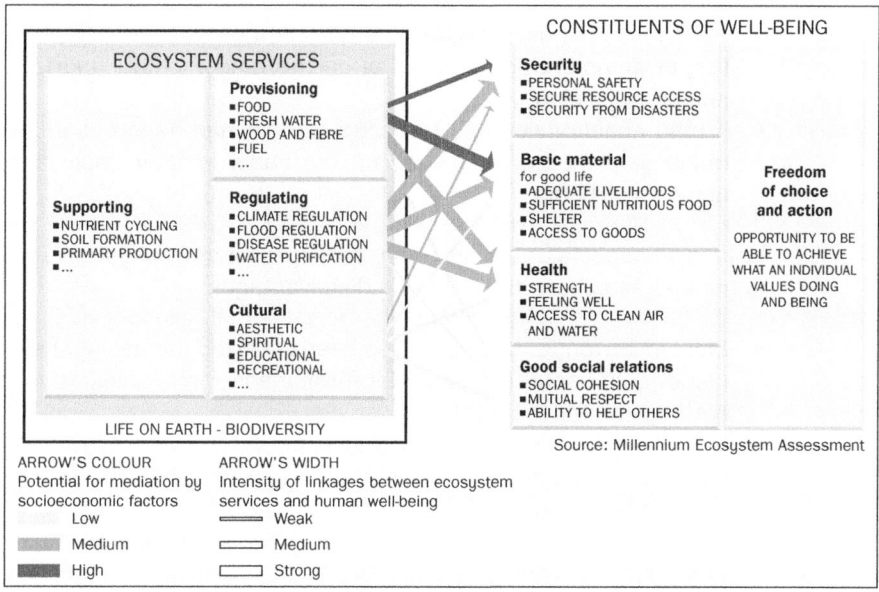

Figure 7.1: Relationships between human populations and their economic and social activities, and the resultant links of the ecosystem with human health and activities

Source: Millennium Assessment Report (2000)

✎ Activity 7.1

Look at Figure 7.1. You will find that there are links between many different factors depicted in this figure. In particular, this conceptual diagram attempts to create links between human well-being and all aspects of the planetary environment. Consider two advantages of the linkage of all aspects of the planetary environment as ecosystem services to humans. Then consider two disadvantages of this linkage.

Feedback

Linking all aspects of the planetary environment as ecosystem services to humans may have the following advantages:

- It may enable us to realize the importance of planetary processes that we do not normally link to our health directly. For example, ordinarily we may appreciate the direct linkage between a provisioning service, such as water, for our health, but we do not normally appreciate the hydrological cycle of the planet that supports availability of this provisioning service.

- It may enable policymakers to argue for the protection of the plane-tary environment on the basis of earth's fundamental importance to human well-being.
- It may enable scientists to document the importance of a broader range of planetary resources on the basis of their importance to human well-being.

Linking all aspects of the planetary environment as ecosystem services to humans may have the following disadvantages:

- Most importantly, the model has been criticized for making the entire planet only useful if it is useful for humans – effectively, this is an anthropocentric model.
- It is also problematic for many scientists that many individual spe-cies and elements of the planetary environment are difficult to link to human well-being.
- You might also consider this from a cultural perspective. Many cul-tures and world religions consider other species and elements of the environment to have equal rights to existence with humans – and not to be important only as ecosystem services for humans.

The risks to human health from global environmental change

The scale of GEC and its many different modes and paths of causal influ-ence on health outcomes represent an important difference from environ-mental concerns that relate to localized toxicological or microbiological hazards to health. While billions of people still suffer from illnesses related to a poor local physical environment, humans, as a species, are also cross-ing a new frontier of potential planetary destruction. In this context, there is a need to understand the range of likely adverse health impacts and other consequences of global environmental changes. This provides chal-lenges for science and policy: for scientists the causal pathways from global change to health impacts are lengthy and complex. For policy, many of these global changes require global responses – in a policy environment organized fundamentally by states and regions (as we explore in Chapter 9), with some decisions made at global level through multilateral decision-making structures such as the UN (see Chapter 10).

Climate change

To date, the most extensive and best developed GEC-related health risk assessments have been done in relation to stratospheric ozone depletion (with its mostly direct-acting risks to skin and eyes) and global climate change. On climate change, the picture is fairly bleak. In 2019, greenhouse gas concentrations reached new record highs of carbon dioxide (CO_2), methane (CH) and nitrous oxide (N_2O) which were, respectively, 148 per cent, 260 per cent and 123 per cent of pre-industrial (before 1750) levels (World Meteorological Organization 2020). There now remains little scientific debate about the relationship between human-generated 'greenhouse gases' and the world's climate system (Cook et al. 2013).

As the global climate changes, there is evidence of changes to regional rainfall patterns, with increases over the oceans but reductions over much of the land surface, especially in various low-to-medium latitude mid-continental regions (central Spain, American mid-west, the Sahel, Amazonia), and in already arid areas in northwest India, the Middle East, northern Africa and parts of Central America. Rainfall events are intensifying with more frequent extreme events increasing the likelihood of flooding and droughts, as we are already witnessing in Europe and in Asia. Regional weather systems, including the great South-West Asian monsoon, could undergo latitudinal shift. Climatologists also note that there will be increasingly severe weather events, including more powerful storms and stronger winds, intensification of the El Niño cycle and altered patterns of drought and rainfall (World Meteorological Organization 2020; Intergovernmental Panel on Climate Change (IPCC) 2021).

With climate change, sea levels are rising, and oceans are warming. Even if the build-up in greenhouse gases is arrested by mid-twenty-first century, the seas will continue to expand as the extra heat permeates the ocean and as on-land glaciers continue to melt at warmer temperatures (World Meteorological Organization 2020). With two-thirds of the world's population living within 60 km of the sea, a rise in sea level would have widespread health impacts. The countries most vulnerable to sea-level rise include Bangladesh and Egypt, with huge river delta farming populations, and Pakistan, Indonesia and Thailand, with large coastal populations. Various low-lying island populations in the Pacific and Indian Oceans face the prospect of wholesale displacement. For example, Jakarta, Indonesia's capital city on the island of Java, is both one of the most densely populated cities in the world, and one of the most threatened by climate change. In 2020, Indonesia announced to the world that its capital would be moved to the island of Borneo (Van de Vuurst and Escobar 2020).

Some of the world's coastal arable land and fish-nurturing mangroves will be damaged by sea-level rise. Rising seas would salinate coastal freshwater aquifers, particularly under small islands. A heightening of storm surges would damage coastal roadways, sanitation systems and housing (World Meteorological Organization 2020).

Stratospheric ozone depletion

Various human-produced industrial gases, especially halogenated compounds (such as the chlorofluorocarbons used for refrigeration and insulated packaging), destroy ozone molecules in the stratosphere. This allows greater penetration to the Earth's surface of solar ultraviolet radiation (UVR), particularly at higher (above approximately 35°) latitudes, including southern Australia, southern South America, Northern Europe and Canada. This increase in UVR exposure increases the risk of skin cancer (malignant melanoma, non-melanocytic cancers). Other risks include an increase in the incidence of ocular cataracts, other eye disorders such as squamous-cell cancer of the conjunctiva and suppression of the immune system (e.g. lower vaccination efficacy, reduced risk of autoimmune disorders) (Velders et al. 2007).

Disruption and degradation of various ecosystems

The increasing human demand for space, materials and food leads to increasingly rapid extinction of populations and species of animals and plants. With processes such as deforestation, whole ecosystems are destroyed. This, in turn, can disrupt ecosystems that provide nature's goods and services, and can impact on global ecosystem stability. Meanwhile, 'invasive' species are spreading into new environments in association with intensified trade, population mobility and food production. These bio-invasions have myriad consequences for health. With these processes the health impacts are indirect – we may lose, before discovery, many natural chemicals and genes with potential medical and health benefits (WHO and CBD 2015; UNEP 2021; WHO 2021).

Impairment of food-producing ecosystems

Increasing pressures from agricultural and livestock production put stresses on arable lands and pastures, and on forests. In the early twenty-first century, it is estimated one-third of the world's previously productive land is adversely affected by erosion, compaction, salinization, waterlogging and chemicalization, which destroy organic content.

Similar pressures on the world's ocean fisheries have left most severely depleted or stressed. The Food and Agriculture Organization (FAO 2020) reports that, despite national attempts to control overfishing, 'the proportion of fish stocks within biologically sustainable levels has continued to decrease, dropping from 90 percent in 1974 to 65.8 percent in 2017' (Food and Agriculture Organization 2020).

Loss of biodiversity

In 2011, a survey of 583 conservation scientists reported an undivided (99.5 per cent) view that 'it is likely a serious loss of biological diversity is underway' and 'many scientists do not fully support the utilitarian concept of ecosystem services' (Rudd 2011: 1165). In the face of massive extinctions and limited funding, conservation scientists debate controversial emergency conservation strategies such as triage, drawing from medicine's emergency procedures to develop means to prioritize species or ecosystems on the basis of their 'utility' (Myers et al. 2000; Parr et al. 2009; Wilson and Law 2016).

Meanwhile, there are many scientists who contend that there is an urgent need to improve understanding of the importance of biodiversity for human health and well-being, some arguing that only an anthropocentric view of biodiversity within a paradigm 'ecosystem service' will enable decision makers to prioritize the theme. This need for understanding is especially urgent in fragile and vulnerable ecosystems where communities depend directly on the resources of their environment (Stephens 2012).

In 2015, WHO and the Convention on Biological Diversity (CBD) published its first state of knowledge review on the importance of biodiversity to human health (WHO and CBD 2015). Even as this advance was underway, the CBD undertook a major review of progress towards protection of biodiversity and showed a massive decline in biodiversity across the world (Leadley et al. 2014). In 2020, WWF and the Institute of Zoology undertook their review of the planet's biodiversity. They found that there has been a catastrophic 68 per cent global decrease in population sizes of mammals, birds, amphibians, reptiles and fish between 1970 and 2016 (WWF 2020). This not only impacts on food sources for humans, but these population crashes combine with extinctions and deplete the genetic diversity of the planet for the future.

It is important to note that the destruction of biodiverse ecosystems internationally is not by communities directly dependent on these ecosystems but from processes such as deforestation, mining, resource extraction and biopiracy, generated by global human demand for products such as timber or for foods such as soya or beef. These processes are also facilitated by trade liberalization (Rodrigues and Almeida 2016). Rich countries and their populations have been particularly responsible for the resource extraction that impacts negatively on biodiversity and on the well-being of local communities. However, increasingly, urban populations in every country demand resources and products from biodiverse regions, and with rising urban populations this threat is likely to increase (UNDP 2020).

Water including wetlands

Freshwater supplies are coming under increasing pressure around the world. Various major (subterranean) aquifers, in all continents, are being depleted. In the world's mid-latitude belts, this is likely to be exacerbated by a decline in rainfall due to climate change – even as rainfall increases and becomes more intense at lower and higher latitudes. Agricultural and industrial demand, amplified by population growth, often greatly exceeds both the rate of natural recharge of aquifers and flow rate within river systems.

With climate change, water stresses are exacerbated: yields of cereal grains are likely to decrease in the tropics where many countries are already under water stress. Drought also leads to forest fires, which have been associated with an increased risk of health impacts such as respiratory disease, eye problems, injuries and fatalities (World Meteorological Organization 2020).

Wetlands are among the world's most productive water environments. They host enormous biological diversity that provides the water and productivity for the survival of innumerable species of plants and animals, and the people who rely on them. They are among the most threatened environments in the world (Ramsar Convention on Wetlands (2021).

Oceans

Oceans are not just important as an ecosystem providing food for billions of people, or as a threat to human health as sea levels rise. There are also other major changes occurring to oceans that affect all marine life and human well-being. As the concentration of CO_2 in the atmosphere rises, so does the concentration of CO_2 in the oceans. This affects ocean chemistry, lowering the average pH of the water, a process known as ocean acidification. This affects many organisms and ecosystem services, threatening food security by endangering marine life. It also affects coastal protection by weakening coral reefs. Oceans are also warming with consequent effects on marine life. Marine heatwaves are also now a significant event with impacts on marine life and on the communities depending on the oceans for food and livelihoods (World Meteorological Organization 2020). Overall, long-term ocean warming, deoxygenation and acidification are also now major problems globally and have significant impacts on marine life, on the communities that rely on the oceans for both their food and livelihoods, and on overall sustainability of the oceans of the world (World Meteorological Organization 2020).

Waste

As we discussed in Chapter 3, urbanization and globalization have made changes all over the world to our social values and material consumption. This in turn has consequences for waste generation. The World Bank calculates, very dramatically, that we could be 'drowning in waste by 2050' (Kaza et al. 2018). The calculations of waste generation are shocking, if we also consider that much waste, particularly plastic and toxic waste, is exported from richer to poorer nations, and then affects the poorest peoples in these countries. This then becomes a major issue for environmental justice (UNEP 2021).

Within waste, plastics, particularly single use plastics, pose an enormous risk to the planet and in mostly indirect ways, to human health and well-being. Plastics also pose a major threat to other species. UNEP estimates that 'from 1950 to 2015, 8.3 billion metric tons of new plastics were produced. Without action, the annual flow of plastic into the ocean will nearly triple by 2040, to 29 million metric tons per year (range: 23 million–37 million metric tons per year), equivalent to 50 kg of plastic per metre of coastline worldwide' (UNEP 2021). This plastic pollution affects the poorest peoples of the world most severely, often in direct ways for waste pickers working in hazardous waste sites and exposed to the chemicals and additives that plastics contain. It also affects the whole planet and there is now overwhelming evidence that micro-plastics have entered the food chain globally (UNEP 2021).

 Activity 7.2

Based on your reading of other chapters so far, list four ways in which globalization is likely to contribute to the occurrence of global changes to our ecosystem services.

Feedback

Globalization might contribute to global environmental change and affect our eco-system service in the following ways:

- Long-distance and rapid trade, discussed in Chapters 2 and 3, accelerates the inadvertent global distribution of 'exotic' species of insects, animals and plants. Some thrive in their new environments, disrupting ecosystems and displacing local food species.
- The intensification and increased corporate control of world food production entail increasing use of energy and nitrogenous fertilizer. This has hugely increased the entry of activated nitrogenous compounds into the environment, changing the global nitrogen cycle and causing significantly altered chemical balance and acidity in waterways and soils.
- As Chapter 2 highlights, the globalization of consumption patterns (in conjunction with rapid urbanization) stimulates GEC. This includes moves to a more globalized diet and links to deforestation to open up pastoral land. Widespread environmental degradation and carbon dioxide emissions result.
- As trade intensifies and spreads, many countries are driven to develop exports to generate foreign exchange. In exploiting their distinctive export opportunities, they may do so in ways that damage the local natural resource base. The widespread occurrence of uncontrolled logging is a well-known example, leading to widespread loss of locally valued forest products, species extinctions, flood control, mobilization of infectious agents (especially viruses) into human communities and release of greenhouse gases.

Health impacts of global environmental changes

There are direct and indirect ways in which GEC can affect human health. Furthermore, some impacts will occur relatively immediately, while others will depend on a succession of changes in natural systems and may occur incrementally. Other GECs affect the fundamental determinants of our health. These include changes to the oceans, the loss of biodiversity globally and the destruction of habitats such as forests and wetlands.

For climate changes, the already emerging direct health impacts include those due to changes in exposure to thermal extremes (heat and cold); increases in extreme weather events (floods, cyclones, storm-surges, droughts); and increased production of certain air pollutants and aero-allergens (spores and moulds). Effects are not evenly spread. Milder winters in temperate countries may reduce the seasonal winter-time mortality peak, but globally the increased frequency of heatwaves may increase summer mortality. WHO estimates that between 2000 and 2016, the number of people exposed to heatwaves increased by around 125 million (WHO 2021). Further increase in temperatures in currently hot regions might impair mosquito survival. However, as average surface temperatures gradually rise, there is an increase in climatic variability. Many scientists consider that human health and safety are more endangered by increases in extreme weather events than by changes in average climate conditions (IPCC 2021).

Climate change, acting via less direct mechanisms, is already affecting regional food productivity (IPCC 2021). This itself is linked to other processes such as deforestation, which not only diminishes the potential future food sources from biodiverse forests but also can lead to unsustainable agricultural practices on resource poor soils. This combines with impacts of climate change on food production.

Deforestation, exacerbated by climate change, affects the transmission of many infectious diseases, especially water-, food- and vector-borne diseases. In the longer term, these indirect impacts are likely to have greater magnitude than more direct impacts (see Chapter 5). Vector-borne infections are of particular relevance. The distribution and abundance of vector organisms and intermediate hosts are affected by physical factors (temperature, precipitation, humidity, surface water and wind) and biotic factors (vegetation, host species, predators, parasites and human interventions). A temperature increase causes net increases, worldwide, in the geographic range of various vector organisms, although some localized decreases might occur. Deforestation exposes new populations to forest vectors.

Extreme weather events such as severe storms, floods and drought have claimed millions of lives since the turn of the century and have adversely affected the lives of many more as well as costing enormous amounts in property damage. Degradation of the local environment can also contribute to vulnerability from flooding. Extreme weather variability impacts injuries, fatalities and the incidence of infectious diseases, often linked to destruction of water and sanitation services. The first decade of the twenty-first century has seen the effects of these processes, particularly affecting the countries least responsible for climate change and least able to manage the disasters (World Meteorological Organization 2020; IPCC 2021). Bangladesh, for example, is ranked sixth among the world's top 10 countries most affected by extreme weather events in the last 20 years, with 70 per cent of its population living in flood-prone regions, with a quarter of these affected by cyclones (Matsuyama et al. 2020).

Sustainability, health and well-being – global policies for GEC

There is growing public appreciation and discussion of the need to achieve sustainable environmental and social development (UNDP and University of Oxford 2021).

Long-term thinking and planning for planetary well-being form the true bottom-line of 'sustainability', with health of humans, but also of other species, as the main criterion. Sustainability will require us to achieve societies able to maintain and live within the limits of the natural resource base and its ecosystems, and to maintain internal social cohesion. As noted earlier, humankind is now overloading the biosphere. One helpful way of visualizing and thinking about this is in relation to our transgressing of critical 'planetary boundaries' (Rockstrom et al. 2009).

The restoration of balance, at global level, between human numbers, demands, waste generation, and the capacity of the planet to supply, replenish and absorb is a huge and worldwide task – of a scale and type not previously undertaken by humankind. It requires great effort and imagination across all levels of society and across all cultures (notwithstanding the historical fact that industrializing and empire-building 'Western' society has largely set this planetary overload process in motion). The task is far too big, complex and electorally threatening to be undertaken by individual governments alone.

This final section summarizes a selection of global policies to address the global environmental changes that we have discussed in the previous sections. It may not be clear from the evidence of GECs and their continued and increasing threats, but the international community has been working tirelessly on international agreements since the 1980s. The United Nations agencies most directly involved include the United Nations Environment Programme (UNEP), the Food and Agriculture Organization (FAO) and UN-Habitat.

Perhaps most importantly, there are now overarching policy goals in terms of climate change. The United Nations Framework Convention on Climate Change (UNFCCC) secretariat (also known as UN Climate Change) is a United Nations entity, signed and formed in 1994, to support the global response to the threat of climate change. The Convention is the parent treaty of the 2015 Paris Agreement and the 1997 Kyoto Protocol

(United Nations Framework Convention on Climate Change 2021). Other global policies include those to protect biodiversity, to protect land degradation and desertification, and to achieve the Sustainable Development Goals put in place following the Millennium Development Goals.

It is important to note that there are also a set of policy instruments internationally for the monitoring of the environmental situation globally and progress towards (or not) achieving sustainability. For example, the Intergovernmental Panel on Climate Change (IPCC) is the United Nations body for assessing the science related to climate change. IPCC scientific reports are also a critical input into global climate change negotiations (IPCC 2021). In 2021 IPCC scientists issued their most categoric report to date, concluding that humanity is at a 'code red'.

For biodiversity, the Convention on Biological Diversity also sets global targets, and measures progress (or not) towards these: the Aichi targets were set in 2010, with all countries to develop a National Biodiversity Strategy and Action Plan and to report on the Aichi targets (Secretariat of the Convention on Biological Diversity 2020). Table 7.1 summarizes a range of global agreements addressing key aspects of GEC.

As Table 7.1 shows, several of these environmental agreements are, in technical terms, legally binding. All the agreements have highly differentiated degrees of enforcement and compliance. The oldest convention, the Ramsar Convention on Wetlands, was signed 50 years ago, yet the Ramsar Convention report on the status of Wetlands in 2018, reported that wetlands continue to decline rapidly with 35 per cent loss of wetlands since the 1970s, putting a quarter of the species reliant on wetlands at risk of extinction (Ramsar Convention on Wetlands 2018).

The Convention on Biological Diversity (CBD) is another international convention, signed by 150 governments at the 1992 Rio Earth Summit and with two globally agreed protocols. The AICHI targets of 2010 to 2020 measured national and international performance against the goals of the CBD. Midway through the decade almost no target had been achieved (Leadley et al. 2014). By the end of the decade, the final evaluation in 2020 was published and widely publicized and lamented: almost none of the targets to protect global biodiversity had been met, except a small increase in awareness of the importance of biodiversity in some countries (Secretariat of the Convention on Biological Diversity 2020).

In this context it is even more sobering to note there that there are no global conventions, let alone legally binding global agreements, for the global protection of forests, or for the global protection of oceans. In the case of forests, there have been decades of debate about a global agreement. In 2000 the Food and Agriculture Organization (FAO) commissioned reports on global governance of forests: in a major analysis, Ruiz reported that there are no global agreements but there are up to 10 specific conventions that deal with aspects of deforestation, including the commodity oriented International Tropical Timber Agreement and associated WTO rules (Ruiz 2001). There is widespread recognition that forests, and trees outside forests, are hugely important for the planet and human well-being, far

Table 7.1 Selected global policies to address global environmental changes

Theme	Policy	Key facts	Full information
Wetlands	Ramsar Convention on Wetlands	The Convention on Wetlands is the oldest of the modern global intergovernmental environmental agreements. It was adopted in the Iranian city of Ramsar in 1971 and came into force in 1975. Since then, almost 90% of UN member states, from all the world's geographic regions, have acceded to become 'Contracting Parties'. Its aim is the conservation and wise use of all wetlands through local and national actions and international cooperation, as a contribution towards achieving sustainable development throughout the world.	https://globalization.ramsar.org
Ozone	The Vienna Convention for the Protection of the Ozone Layer	The Vienna Convention was the first convention of any kind to be signed by all countries, taking effect in 1988 and reaching universal ratification in 2009. This agreement is a framework convention that lays out principles to protect the ozone layer. It does not require countries to take control actions to protect the ozone layer.	https://ozone.unep.org/treaties/vienna-convention
Ozone	The Montreal Protocol on Substances that Deplete the Ozone Layer	The Montreal Protocol is a global agreement, linked to the Vienna Convention to protect the Earth's ozone layer by phasing out the chemicals that deplete it. This phase-out plan includes both the production and consumption of ozone-depleting substances (particularly CFCs). The agreement was signed in 1987 and entered into force in 1989. In 2019, the Kigali Amendment entered into force to also reduce the production of hydrofluorocarbons (HFCs) (which had been adopted in some countries after the phasing out of CFCs) due to the powerful greenhouse gas emissions and contribution to climate change of HFCs.	https://ozone.unep.org/treaties/montreal-protocol
Climate Change	United Nations Framework Convention on Climate Change	The UNFCCC entered into force on 21 March 1994. In 2021, it has near-universal membership and 197 countries have ratified the Convention. Its aim is to prevent 'dangerous' human interference with the climate system.	https://unfccc.int
Climate Change	The Kyoto Protocol	The Kyoto Protocol operationalizes the UNFCCC by committing 37 industrialized countries and economies in transition to limit and reduce greenhouse gas (GHG) emissions in accordance with agreed individual targets. It was adopted on 11 December 1997. Notably it did not place any obligations on any other countries. It finally entered into force on 16 February 2005. In 2021, there are 192 Parties to the Kyoto Protocol.	https://unfccc.int/kyoto_protocol

(Continued)

Table 7.1 (Continued)

Theme	Policy	Key facts	Full information
Climate Change	The Paris Agreement	The Paris Agreement is a legally binding agreement signed by 196 countries in 2015. Its goal is to limit global warming to well below 2, preferably to 1.5 degrees Celsius, compared to pre-industrial levels. It was adopted by 196 Parties at COP 21 in Paris, on 12 December 2015 and entered into force on 4 November 2016. In 2021, 191 Parties have ratified the agreement. Notably, all countries commit to take action under the Paris Agreement.	https://unfccc.int/ process-and-meetings/the-paris-agreement/ the-paris-agreement
Biodiversity	The Convention on Biological Diversity (CBD)	The Convention on Biological Diversity was signed by 150 governments at the 1992 Rio Earth Summit. It entered into force in 1993. It has three aims: the conservation of biological diversity; the sustainable use of the components of biological diversity; and the fair and equitable sharing of the benefits arising out of the utilization of genetic resources.	https:// globalization.cbd.int
Biodiversity	CBD Cartagena Protocol on Biosafety	The Cartagena Protocol was adopted in 2000 and entered into force in 2003. This agreement aims to ensure the safe handling, transport and use of living modified organisms (LMOs) resulting from modern biotechnology that may have adverse effects on biological diversity, taking also into account risks to human health.	http://bch.cbd.int/ protocol
Biodiversity	CBD Nagoya Protocol on Access to Genetic Resources and the Fair and Equitable Sharing of Benefits Arising from their Utilization	This Nagoya Protocol aims at sharing the benefits arising from the utilization of genetic resources in a fair and equitable way. It entered into force on 12 October 2014. It operationalizes the third objective of the CBD. The Nagoya Protocol also covers traditional knowledge (TK) associated with genetic resources that are covered by the CBD and the benefits arising from its utilization. It sets out core obligations for its contracting Parties to take measures in relation to access to genetic resources, benefit-sharing and compliance.	https:// globalization.cbd. int/abs/
Desertification	The United Nations Convention to combat Desertification	Signed by 174 governments, the UNCD entered into force in 1996. It is the sole legally binding international agreement focused on sustainable land management, specifically in the arid, semi-arid and dry sub-humid areas, known as the drylands of the planet.	https:// globalization.unccd. int

beyond their value as timber (Food and Agriculture Organization 2018). A special UN Forum on Forests exists for the follow-up and review of the implementation of the United Nations Strategic Plan for Forests 2030 (United Nations Department of Economic and Social Affairs and United Nations Forum on Forests Secretariat 2021).

In the case of oceans, there are multiple regional agreements and national agreements related to management of seas and fisheries around specific countries. However, the key issue for the protection of oceans is related to the vast ocean areas known as Areas Beyond National Jurisdiction (ABNJ) which make up an astonishing 45 per cent of the Earth's surface. These ABNJ have few laws to protect their exploitation (International Union for the Conservation of Nature 2021).

It is important to note that there is truly positive evidence of the value of global concerted action, and that this can be done by governments coming together through these agreements. For example, the Montreal Protocol has been lauded as the most successful environmental treaty to date. The protocol has been extremely successful in its original aim of cutting production and use of chlorofluorocarbons (CFCs) and other ozone-depleting substances, with nearly 99 per cent of ozone-depleting substances phased-out by its 30 year anniversary of 2017. A 2019 analysis found that 'without the Montreal Protocol, UVI values at northern and southern latitudes <50° would by now be 10 to 20% larger in all seasons compared to UVIs observed during the early 1990s . . . for latitudes >50°S, UVI values would have increased over the same period between 25% (Ushuaia in summer and autumn) to more than 100% (South Pole in spring and summer)' (McKenzie et al. 2019).

Multilateral actors such as the United Nations can also advance policies on GEC independently. UN-Habitat has worked since the late 1980s on collating evidence from towns and cities globally on local policies that work towards sustainable urbanization (UN-Habitat 2020). As we noted in Chapter 3, it is highly significant that UNDP, in 2020, for the first time ever, now include a measure of a country's population impact on the planet, in its ground-breaking Human Development Index (HDI) – 30 years after the first HDI was launched to add social aspects of development to measures of human progress (UNDP 2020). Individual governments have a strong role also: in 2021 the UNEP and World Resources Institute (2021) produced a clear legislative guide aimed at individual countries for the regulation of single-use plastic products, recognizing that state governments have an important role to play in controlling the production of this waste. Civil society – all of us – have an equally important role to take.

Summary

Globalization has become a reality of the twenty-first century, and – given ongoing population growth and the extensification and intensification of economic activity (much of it based on fossil fuel combustion) – global environmental changes are an entrenched reality of today and the future. It is important to monitor global environmental change and its impacts on health and to relate estimates of health risks more directly to policy and social decision-making. This should be done globally, regionally, nationally and locally.

You have seen how the impacts of global environmental change are complex, how they affect the climate, agricultural production, water, biodiversity, oceans and forests, each of which in turn has an impact on health. You have seen a selection of the global agreements and actions that attempt to lead us towards a more sustainable future.

References

Abman, R. and Lundberg, C. (2020) Does free trade increase deforestation? The effects of regional trade agreements, *Journal of the Association of Environmental and Resource Economists*, 7(1). Available at: https://doi.org/10.1086/705787.

Cook, J., Nuccitelli, Green, S., Richardson, M. et al. (2013) Quantifying the consensus on anthropogenic global warming in the scientific literature, *Environmental Research Letters*, 8: 024024. Available at: https://doi.org/10.1088/1748-9326/8/2/024024 (accessed 5 May 2021).

Food and Agriculture Organization (FAO) (2018) Forests and sustainable cities, *Unasylva: An International Journal of Forestry and Forest Industries*, 69(2018/1). Available at: http://globalization.fao.org/3/I8707EN/i8707en.pdf (accessed 15 June 2021).

Food and Agriculture Organization (FAO) (2020) Tracking progress on food and agriculture-related SDG indicators 2020: a report on the indicators under FAO custodianship. Available at: http://globalization.fao.org/sdg-progress-report/en/ (accessed 30 May 2021).

Intergovernmental Panel on Climate Change (IPCC) (2021) *Climate Change 2021: The Physical Science Basis. Contribution of Working Group I to the Sixth Assessment Report of the Intergovernmental Panel on Climate Change* [V. Masson-Delmotte, P. Zhai, A. Pirani et al. (eds.)]. Cambridge: Cambridge University Press. In Press.

International Union for the Conservation of Nature (IUCN) (2021) International ocean governance. Available at: https://globalization.iucn.org/theme/marine-and-polar/our-work/international-ocean-governance (accessed 30 May 2021).

Kaza, S., Yao, L.C., Bhada-Tata, P. et al. (2018) *What a Waste 2.0: A Global Snapshot of Solid Waste Management to 2050*. Urban Development; Washington, DC: World Bank. Available at: https://openknowledge.worldbank.org/handle/10986/30317 (accessed 30 May 2021)

Leadley, P., Krug, C.B., Alkemade, R. et al. (2014) *Progress towards the Aichi Biodiversity Targets: An Assessment of Biodiversity Trends, Policy Scenarios and Key Actions*. Montreal, Canada: Secretariat of the Convention on Biological Diversity, Technical Series 78. Available at: https://globalization.cbd.int/doc/publications/cbd-ts-78-en.pdf (accessed 2 May 2021).

Lewis, S. and Maslin, M. (2015) Defining the Anthropocene, *Nature*, 519: 171–180. Available at: https://doi.org/10.1038/nature14258.

Matsuyama, A., Khan, F.A. and Khalequzzaman, M. (2020) Bangladesh Public health issues and implications to flood risk reduction, in E. Chan and R. Shaw (eds) *Public Health and Disasters. Disaster Risk Reduction (Methods, Approaches and Practices)*. Singapore: Springer.

McKenzie, R., Bernhard, G., Liley, B. et al. (2019) Success of Montreal Protocol demonstrated by comparing high-quality UV measurements with 'world avoided' calculations from two chemistry-climate models, *Nature Scientific Reports*, 9: 12332. Available at: https://doi.org/10.1038/s41598-019-48625-z.

McMichael, A. (1993) *Planetary Overload: Global Environmental Change and the Health of the Human Species.* Cambridge: Cambridge University Press.

Millennium Assessment Report (2000) Graphic resources. Available at: http://globalization.millenniumassessment.org/en/GraphicResources.aspx (accessed 5 May 2021).

Myers, N., Mittermeier, R.A., Mittermeier, C.G. et al. (2000) Biodiversity hotspots for conservation priorities, *Nature*, 403(6772): 853–858.

Parr, M.J., Bennun, L., Boucher, T. et al. (2009) Why we should aim for zero extinction, *Trends in Ecology and Evolution*, 24(4): 181; author reply 183–184.

Ramsar Convention on Wetlands (2018) *Global Wetland Outlook: State of the World's Wetlands and their Services to People.* Gland, Switzerland: Ramsar Convention Secretariat. Available at: https://globalization.ramsar.org/sites/default/files/documents/library/gwo_e.pdf (accessed 17 June 2021).

Ramsar Convention on Wetlands (2021) The importance of wetlands, Ramsar Convention on Wetlands. Available at: https://globalization.ramsar.org/about/the-importance-of-wetlands (accessed 15 June 2021).

Rockstrom, J., Steffen, W. and Noone, K. (2009) A safe operating space for humanity, *Nature*, 461: 472–475.

Rodrigues, W. and Almeida, A. (2016) Relationship between openness to trade and deforestation: empirical evidence from the Brazilian Amazon, *Ecological Economics*, 121: 85–97. Available at: https://doi.org/10.1016/j.ecolecon.2015.11.014.

Rudd, M.A. (2011) Scientists' opinions on the global status and management of biological diversity, *Conservation Biology*, 25(6): 1165–1175.

Ruiz, B. (2001) No forest convention but ten tree treaties. In special edition global conventions related to forests, *Unasylva: an International Journal of Forestry and Forest Industries*, 52(2001/3). Available at: http://globalization.fao.org/3/y1237e/y1237e03.htm#P0_0 (accessed 29 May 2021).

Secretariat of the Convention on Biological Diversity (2020) *Global Biodiversity Outlook 5.* Montreal. Available at: https://globalization.cbd.int/gbo/gbo5/publication/gbo-5-en.pdf (accessed 30 May 2021).

Stephens, C. (2012) Biodiversity and global health: hubris, humility and the unknown, *Environmental Research Letters*, 7(1): 011008.

UNDP (2020) *Human Development Report 2020: The Next Frontier. Human Development and the Anthropocene*, United Nations Development Programme. Available at: http://hdr.undp.org/sites/default/files/hdr2020.pdf (accessed 18 May 2021).

UNDP and University of Oxford (2021) *People's Climate Vote*. New York and Oxford: United Nations Development Programme and University of Oxford. Available at: https://globalization.undp.org/content/dam/undp/library/km-qap/UNDP-Oxford-Peoples-Climate-Vote-Results.pdf (accessed 17 May 2021).

United Nations Department of Economic and Social Affairs (UNDESA) (2019) *United Nations Population Division. World Population Prospects: 2019 Revision.* New York: United Nations Department of Economic and Social Affairs. Available at: https://population.un.org/wpp/ (accessed 27 April 2021).

United Nations Department of Economic and Social Affairs, United Nations Forum on Forests Secretariat (2021) *The Global Forest Goals Report 2021.* Available at: *globalization.un.org/esa/forests* (accessed 1 May 2021.)

United Nations Framework Convention on Climate Change (2021) *The Paris Agreement.* Available at: https://unfccc.int/process-and-meetings/the-paris-agreement/the-paris-agreement (accessed 1 May 2021).

UNEP (2021) *Neglected: Environmental Justice Impacts of Marine Litter and Plastic Pollution*. Available at: https://wedocs.unep.org/xmlui/bitstream/handle/20.500.11822/35417/EJIPP.pdf (accessed 20 May 2021).

UNEP and World Resources Institute (2021) *Tackling Plastic Pollution: Legislative Guide for the Regulation of Single-Use Plastic Products.* Available at: https://wedocs.unep.org/bitstream/handle/20.500.11822/34570/PlastPoll.pdf.pdf?sequence=3&isAllowed=globalization (accessed 10 June 2021).

UNEP-GEAS (2012) One planet, how many people? A review of Earth's carrying capacity. Discussion Paper for the Year of Rio+20. Available at: http://na.unep.net/geas/archive/pdfs/GEAS_Jun_12_Carrying_Capacity.pdf (accessed 20 May 2021).

UN-Habitat (2020) *World Cities Report 2020: The Value of Sustainable Urbanization*. Nairobi: UN-Habitat. Available at: https://unhabitat.org/World%20Cities%20Report%202020 (accessed 2 May 2021).

Van de Vuurst, P. and Escobar, L. (2020) Perspective: climate change and the relocation of Indonesia's capital to Borneo, *Frontiers in Earth Science*, 8. Available at: https://globalization.frontiersin.org/article/10.3389/feart.2020.00005 (accessed 15 June 2021).

Velders, G., Andersen, S., Daniel, J. et al. (2007) The importance of the Montreal Protocol in protecting climate, *Proceedings of the National Academy of Sciences* 104(12): 4814–4819. Available at: https://doi.org/10.1073/pnas.0610328104.

Venter, O., Sanderson, E., Magrach, A. et al. (2016) Sixteen years of change in the global terrestrial human footprint and implications for biodiversity conservation. *Nature Communications*, 7: 12558. Available at: https://doi.org/10.1038/ncomms12558 (accessed 8 May 2021).

Wilson, K. and Law, E. (2016) Ethics of conservation triage, *Frontiers in Ecology and Evolution*, (4)112. Available at: https://doi.org/10.3389/fevo.2016.00112 (accessed 12 May 2021).

World Health Organization (2021) Heatwaves. Available at: https://globalization.who.int/health-topics/heatwaves#tab=tab_1 (accessed 15 June 2021).

World Health Organization (WHO) and Convention on Biological Diversity (CBD) (2015) *Connecting Global Priorities: Biodiversity and Human Health – a State of Knowledge Review.* Available at: https://globalization.who.int/publications/i/item/connecting-global-priorities-biodiversity-and-human-health (accessed 3 May 2021).

World Health Organization (WHO) and Regional Office for Europe (2021) Nature, biodiversity and health: an overview of interconnections, World Health Organization. Regional Office for Europe. Available at: https://apps.who.int/iris/handle/10665/341376 (accessed 6 June 2021).

World Meteorological Organization (2020) *State of the World Global Climate 2020 WMO-1264*. Available at: https://library.wmo.int/doc_num.php?explnum_id=10618 (accessed 5 May 2021).

WWF (2020) Almond, R.E.A., Grooten M. and Petersen, T. (eds) (2020) *Living Planet Report 2020 – Bending the curve of biodiversity loss*. Gland, Switzerland: WWF. Available at: https://globalization.wwf.org.uk/sites/default/files/2020-09/LPR20_Full_report.pdf (accessed 5 January 2021).

Global health and security

Preslava Stoeva

8

Overview

This chapter critically examines the links between the field of security and global health issues. It begins with an introduction to the concept of security and the key debates surrounding how security is defined before exploring the links between global health and security and the ways in which specific threats to health have been framed as threats to security.

Learning objectives

After working through this chapter, you will be able to:

- Describe multiple ways in which security can be conceptualized.
- Explain how and why health and security interface.
- Critically reflect on the differences between defining health as a national security and a human security issue.
- Recognize how different health-related threats have received attention from the security community.
- Understand the benefits and risks of linking global health with a security agenda.

Key terms

Health security: The concern with and activities associated with the impact of diseases and other health-related concerns across state borders, which endanger the life and well-being of individuals and communities, but also impact the stability and prosperity of states.

Human Security: A concern with individual life and human dignity, involving safety from such chronic threats as hunger, disease and repression, and protection from sudden and hurtful disruptions in the patterns of daily life (UNDP 1994).

International Relations (IR): A social science discipline, which examines the relations between states, their interactions within formal and informal international organizations, as well as more recently the transborder work of a broad range of non-state actors. The discipline is subdivided into various fields with a narrower focus – e.g. international relations theory, global governance, security studies, development studies, international political economy, international law and so on.

National security: The defence of the state against military and other types of serious threats to its sovereignty, integrity and core values.

Defining security

Security is a central concept in the study of international politics. Mainstream international relations theories maintain that security is the primary consideration of states as they interact in the international system. The definition and scope of security are, however, contested. Williams and McDonald (2018) argue that four fundamental questions define the field of inquiry: what is security?; security for whom?; security from what?; and security by what means? (e.g. military, economic, social, etc.).

What is security?

In the field of international politics, security has most often been defined as the ability of states to maintain their independence and protect their core values and functional integrity (Buzan 1991: 16–19). Security, Buzan argues, is about survival and *freedom from threat*. The solution to security problems, therefore, is deemed to be achievable through military capabilities and through security and defence alliances between states. Such state-centric concepts perceive security in binary terms – states are either secure or they are not. They also view security as a 'zero-sum game' – if one state is secure, another cannot be, which is then seen as a key reason for conflictual and competitive state relations. Threats to security are considered so vital ('high politics') that governments are granted extraordinary powers to use any means necessary to achieve security. Such a conceptualization of security is defined by a narrow scope of security threats and, exceptionalist state- and military-centric thinking.

An alternative way to conceptualize security is to consider it as having a much broader meaning, such as protection from intrusion or attack, individual safety, safety from the indeterminate actions of others (McSweeney 1999: 13). In addition to the traditional conceptualization of security as 'freedom from' (a 'negative freedom'), McSweeney proposes a conceptualization of security as 'freedom to' (a 'positive freedom'). This way of thinking about security is adopted by critical security studies, which argue that people feel secure when they feel they can make choices in their daily lives and that security is about emancipation and empowerment (Booth 2007). Security can therefore be seen as a win-win scenario, where the security of some enhances the security of all. Security politics can then be de-escalated and viewed as everyday politics and approaches to promoting security can take a broad range of forms – economic assistance, cooperation, knowledge-sharing, etc.

Security for whom?

Debates about definitions of security are fundamentally linked to debates about the referent object of security (in short 'the object of security') – in answer to the question 'security for whom?'. Theories of security emerging from the sub-fields of national security studies, strategic (war) studies and from mainstream (principally realist and neo-realist) IR theory envisage the state as the primary referent of security. They argue that the security of the state is a precondition for the security of its inhabitants. When security is defined in this way, health concerns only matter to the extent that they undermine state security (e.g. emerging infectious diseases, new strands or drug-resistant variants of established diseases). The security and survival of the state is pursued by means of foreign and national security policy and eliminating threats to *national security* is perceived as the most important strategic priority for national governments. This perspective, known as *realpolitik*, assumes that state relations are defined by conflict and states' competition for power and domination. A national security approach tends to result in the pursuit of narrow national interests often to the exclusion of the interests of other states or people, in immediate mobilization of resources to address acute threats, in constructing threats as emanating from 'outside' and as being perpetrated by 'others'. This approach eschews any notion of collective security – the idea that security of individual states can be increased through mutually beneficial common action that increases security throughout the international system.

Making the individual the object of security is a central tenet of critical security and *human security* studies. The changing nature of violent conflicts after the end of the Cold War from conflicts between states to conflicts within states, prompted analysts to reconsider the causes of violent conflicts. A new paradigm began to emerge that individual insecurity generated by ethnic tensions, poverty, resource scarcity/abundance and/or economic insecurity drove groups in certain contexts to resort to violence, leading to internal conflict, instability and even state failure (Brainard and Chollet 2007; Collier 2008) as illustrated by the conflicts in Somalia (1993), Rwanda (1994) and Former Yugoslavia (1995). These changes in the nature of conflict prompted a shift in focus in the thinking about security, away from the state to the individual and the threats to individual life and well-being.

The 1994 United Nations Development Programme (UNDP) *Human Development Report* 'New Dimensions of Health Security' argues:

> *The concept of security has for too long been interpreted narrowly: as security of territory from external aggression, or as protection of national interests in foreign policy, or as global security from the threat of nuclear holocaust . . . Forgotten were the legitimate concerns of ordinary people who sought security in their daily lives. For many of them, security symbolized protection from the threat of disease, hunger, unemployment, crime, social conflict, political repression and environmental hazards.*

As Chapters 5 and 6 show, further evidence to support UNDP's argument can be found in the World Health Organization's (WHO) data on the 10 most common causes of death worldwide, which are predominantly communicable and non-communicable diseases linked to the threats identified by UNDP, rather than political conflict or inter-state violence (WHO 2020). Putting individual and community health and well-being at the heart of strategic security politics, however, requires a complete rethink of security policy and practice. A cosmopolitan approach to health as advocated by Brown and Stoeva (2015) provides one example of what this might entail: attention to structural conditions and determinants of health, the pursuit of health equity and justice, transborder responsibility for basic health satisfaction and most importantly a focus on prevention as opposed to short-term response to crises.

Security from what?

Identifying what counts as a security threat is the basis for deciding what means are necessary to address it and this in turn depends on what you consider security to be and who or what needs protecting (i.e. the object of security).

State-centred security approaches define threats to security as any threat to the survival, core values and functional integrity of the state. As such, threats are perceived to be external (i.e. arising from 'outside' the state), caused by other states and military in nature. The changing nature of conflict after the end of the Cold War, however, has demonstrated that insecurity can also be caused by internal factors and by non-state actors. As discussed in the previous section, if security policy is aimed at protecting first the state and then people and collectivities, then threats would be defined as large scale, acute in character, having a destabilizing effect to the normal functioning of the state. Threats could therefore be military but could also stem from a natural disaster, civil conflict or large-scale violence, as well as communicable disease outbreaks with high morbidity and mortality rates.

If, however, security policy is aimed at protecting people and communities first, then the spectrum of threats to security immediately expands to other areas, which some may argue have been neglected or insufficiently addressed. For example, people and communities are threatened by loss of livelihoods from long-term environmental degradation or pollution (see Chapter 7). Poorer and marginalized communities are most often the first ones to be affected and are likely to be affected more profoundly, as they often lack the resources to move to safer, cleaner areas. Poorer and marginalized individuals and communities are much more likely to be affected by, and die prematurely from, non-communicable diseases too (WHO 2021a) (see Chapters 5 and 6). Non-communicable diseases have been an additional risk factor in the Covid-19 pandemic, so preventing NCDs, addressing structural, socio-economic determinants of health as well as ensuring universal access to primary healthcare should be considered strategic priorities for action by states (see Chapter 6). Addressing these would promote both positive ('security to') and negative ('security from') security for individuals and communities.

Security by what means?

The question about how security could be achieved is closely related to the previous three questions about the definition of security, the objects of security and the nature of relevant security threats. A focus on the individual as an object, threatened by diseases or environmental degradation would call for a different set of means to address these threats than a state-centric conceptualization of security, where sources of insecurity are other states and their military capabilities. Strategies to address 'traditional' threats could be said to be fairly straightforward – seeking allies, increasing (military) capabilities, keeping threats 'out'. The growing number of intra-state conflicts and associated consequences – increasing regional instability, migrant flows, political, economic and social collapse of states – make the question of how to achieve or sustain security more challenging. In its first European Union Security Strategy (2003), which established the main principles for advancing the EU's security interests and remains fully relevant, the European Union argued that conflicts can be diffused and avoided altogether and security enhanced by facilitating economic development, growth and better governance, instead of using traditional military methods. This strategy set intentions for a novel approach to addressing security threats by means of seeking transborder, long-term, sustainable, cooperative solutions, in stark contrast with the US security-seeking approach.

In summary, there are four fundamental questions that define the field of security studies and the concept of security: the meaning of security, the object of security, the nature of security threats and the means necessary to pursue and achieve security. Answers to these questions are interrelated and inter-dependent and constitute the working assumptions of our chosen approach to security. The lens through which we see security determines the approaches we privilege for the achievement of our preferred security objectives.

The interface between health and security

Health has traditionally been deemed an issue of 'low politics', in contrast with foreign, defence or economic policy, for example, which would more readily occupy the 'high-politics' agenda. Garrett (1996) and the Institute of Medicine (IOM 1997) identify the potential of health-related challenges to impact on national security and US national interests and advocate therefore that it be placed on the 'high politics' agenda. They argued that emerging and re-emerging infectious diseases could have serious implications for national security by destabilizing the US internally. The argument put forward was as follows – trade liberalization is leading to increased interactions of people, goods and services from different parts of the world, microbes and bacteria are mutating, new diseases are emerging, while investment in disease surveillance and new drugs is dwindling, thus creating the conditions for a 'perfect storm' of uncontrollable spread of pathogens across borders. Diseases could reverse years of economic development or create national and regional instability causing states to fail or descend into conflict (Price-Smith 2009). Fidler (2003) provides detailed analysis of the practical ways in which the linkages between public health and national security have emerged and summarizes the three main concerns that dominated health-related national security agendas in the early 2000s: acute and severe infectious diseases of epidemic potential, HIV/AIDs and bioterrorism. This national security framing of health has been criticized for being dangerously narrow and skewing the security agenda towards a narrow set of threats, as will be discussed in the next section.

Feldbaum and Lee (2004) define a health security risk as any public health issue fitting the following parameters – the issue is of concern to population rather than individual health; it causes high incidence of morbidity/mortality, it has an acute character and cross-border transmission (Feldbaum and Lee 2004). This has affected the ways in which responses to health security threats have been formulated to date – disease-specific, short-term, interventionist, preferencing issues of concern to high-income states. These are some of the characteristics of colonial public health, as discussed in Chapter 4, which entrench health inequities, ignore the health priorities of local populations and create weak health systems dependent on ad-hoc funding and external donors (Holst 2020; Shamasunder et al. 2020).

Health and the human security agenda

In contrast to a narrow national security approach, the 1994 UNDP Human Development Report identified poor health as a threat to human security – a position reaffirmed by the Report of the Commission on Human Security (2003), which further argued that violence, infectious diseases and poverty are the three health challenges that critically impact human security as they affect the vital core values of survival, dignity and livelihood. The significance of human security was reaffirmed by UN General Assembly resolution 66/290 in 2012, which further noted the responsibility of governments to protect and promote the well-being of their citizens and of the international community in complementing this role. One issue with this formulation is that it maintains the centrality of the state both as the main mechanism to address threats to human security (even though states may sometimes be the very source of such insecurity) and to preference the security of some individuals over others (which does not address internal and often politically motivated oppression or marginalization of particular groups of individuals).

These are early signs of how practice is shifting ways of thinking about security. In seeking to assist governments in operationalizing this approach, the UN produced the *Human Security Handbook* (2016), which offers a discussion of the added value of a human security approach and some practical guidance on how to embed a human security perspective in activities towards the realization of the Sustainable Development Goals. In other words, in contrast to conceptualizations of health as a traditional threat to national security (defined in relation to the state and associated with state vulnerability or instability), threats posed by ill-health can also be seen as a threat to the security of individuals and communities in their own right and not just in relation to the security of the state. There are significant benefits in adopting this approach, as it enables a much broader range of health-related issues to fall within the remit of security politics and receive priority attention and resources.

A focus on the security of individuals and communities provides a starting point for a fundamental rethink of the concept of security, of security politics and the means necessary to prevent and address known threats to human life. A human-centred approach to health security, which is sensitive to the needs of diverse individuals and communities within and across states could also support moves to decolonize global health, with a view to shift the focus of health-related security concerns away from the national security interests of powerful states, towards more relevant local health concerns and priorities. A human-centred approach to health security promotes both 'security from' and 'security to', thus supporting not just survival but empowerment and emancipation.

Contemporary health security challenges

The range of health-related challenges to security depends on assumptions made about who it is that is to be made secure. This section briefly introduces three examples – emerging and re-emerging communicable diseases of pandemic potential, non-communicable diseases and health challenges emerging from state insecurity, which illustrate the complexity and inter-connectedness of individual, community and state security.

Emerging and re-emerging communicable diseases of pandemic potential

Although emerging and re-emerging communicable diseases of pandemic potential were framed as one of the key threats to security defined as national security (Fidler 2003; Price-Smith 2009), the Covid-19 pandemic illustrates the continued relevance of this security challenge, albeit for reasons that may be different from earlier justifications. The Covid-19 pandemic has demonstrated the scale of suffering and disruption that infectious diseases can inflict on humanity. It has exposed inequities, interdependencies and interconnectedness within and between societies, as well as weaknesses and inadequacies in pandemic preparedness, health systems resilience and inter-state cooperation. It has prompted WHO Director General Dr Ghebreyesus to remark repeatedly that 'global health security is only as strong as its weakest link and no one is safe until we are all safe' (WHO 2021b). Emerging and re-emerging communicable diseases can be framed as threatening individual, community and state security, to different degrees and with different effects on each of these referent objects. No previous example of a communicable disease epidemic or pandemic has drawn such sharp attention to the need to move beyond short-term, disease-specific interventions, and to start thinking about the need for cooperative, transborder, politically sanctioned action, for strengthening health systems, for developing capacity, resilience and preparedness, for thinking about prevention and conceiving of health security in medium- and long-term time frames. These considerations have more traditionally been associated with the provision of primary healthcare, non-communicable diseases, maternal and child health – areas that are only just beginning to be considered as relevant in some way to the health security problem.

Non-communicable diseases

As discussed in Chapter 6, non-communicable diseases are of chronic, long-term character and cause high levels of morbidity and mortality – around 71 per cent of all global deaths, amounting to around 41 million people each year (WHO 2021a) – and are responsible for a significant percentage of 'premature' deaths. However, they have traditionally not been conceptualized as a threat to health security. For example, according to Feldbaum and Lee's (2004) conceptualization of health-security threats discussed earlier, NCDs do not fall neatly within this category. While the impact of NCDs is primarily on individual health, the long-term treatment of NCDs may have implications for population health, as it requires sizeable resources and puts a significant strain on health systems. NCDs have a significant impact on the well-being and livelihood not only of those directly affected but also on their families, carers and communities. The morbidity and mortality associated with NCDs is very high, as noted earlier, and while NCDs are long term in character, they constitute a risk factor for premature death. NCDs do not constitute a cross-border risk, as they are mostly non-transmissible, but may have transborder origins (e.g. multinational food companies, tobacco and alcohol producers). So, although non-communicable diseases do not fit neatly into a traditional health security framing, we have seen they pose the most significant threat to individual survival, particularly to disadvantaged and marginalized individuals and communities. This example illustrates the argument above that narrow conceptualizations of security obscure relevant threats to the health security of individuals and communities.

✏ Activity 8.1

Read the following two articles:

* Saha, A. and Alleyne, G. (2018) Recognizing noncommunicable diseases as a global health security threat, *Bulletin of the World Health Organisation*, 96: 792–793.
* Lal, A., Erondu, N.A., Heymann, D.L. et al. (2021) Fragmented health systems in Covid-19: rectifying the misalignment between global health security and universal health coverage, *The Lancet*, 397: 61–67.

Is there overlap in the conceptualization of health security and the solutions proposed in these two articles? What are the key differences? Does the article on Covid-19 depart from other articles looking at the relationship between health security and communicable diseases with epidemic potential (see, for example, Fidler 2003)?

Feedback

Look for the ways in which health security is defined in these two articles. What solutions are proposed by the authors? Consider the similarities and differences both of the arguments made and the expected results. There are significant similarities in the proposed approaches, even though they are focusing on two very different threats to health. Can you relate these back to debates about what health issues are considered relevant to security and solutions proposed in earlier discussions of communicable diseases as threats to security?

Delivering emergency and routine health services in conflict settings

Issues that emerge from delivering emergency and routine health services in conflict settings provide an even clearer example of the complex relationship between security and health. This context epitomizes the interconnectedness between the security of individuals, communities and states, and the complex ways in which these inter-relate and co-determine one another. Causality of insecurity flows in multiple ways, re-enforcing the insecurity of all. Conflict settings represent a state of insecurity for the affected state, which can evolve into state fragility and even failure. These settings generate insecurity both for those involved in direct fighting (both individuals and groups) and civilians – who can become intended or unintended targets of attack but also whose inability to access routine healthcare immediately puts them at risk of a broad range of diseases and conditions. Conflict settings represent a threat to healthcare providers as well, as evidenced by increasing reports of attacks on healthcare humanitarian workers and facilities (Dewachi et al. 2014; Stoddard et al. 2020). Conflict, much like a pandemic, disrupts preventive and routine healthcare and public health activities – e.g. vaccination campaigns, maternal and child health, treatment of chronic conditions, primary assessment for non-communicable diseases and public health functions such as water and sanitation (see, for example, Quinn et al. 2017). Conflict overwhelms and disrupts health systems and public health functions, not only by targeting medical personnel, but also by targeting or destroying healthcare infrastructure, disrupting health and public health systems, and increasing the need for emergency and rehabilitative medical services. Individual health security in the context of state insecurity, therefore, is an even more complex problem at the intersection between national and human security.

Benefits and drawbacks of linking health and security

The characterization of global health issues as security threats has generated increased political attention and funding to address some communicable diseases. It has arguably allowed considerable scaling up of some global health activities and initiatives and has led to significantly more attention and resources being directed towards these (Fidler 2003; Rushton 2011). Recognizing health as a threat to the security of individuals and communities, and (only) by extension, states has signalled that it is possible to at least partially reframe security to focus on empowering and emancipating those who are structurally and negatively affected by social, economic and political determinants of health. Bringing health concerns onto the agenda of security politics, in other words, has transformative potential. It can be a catalyst to reframing the way we think about the very definition of security, the values that underpin everyday governance and politics, and focus collective attention on protecting and improving individual lives.

However, the benefits of linking health and security have been questioned for practical and ethical reasons. Concerns have been raised about the potential negative consequences of securitizing health. Thus, Peterson (2002) and McInnes (2011) argue that there is no empirical evidence that infectious diseases in general and HIV/AIDS in particular were capable of destabilizing states or leading to military conflict, but framing these as threats to security had the potential of triggering exceptional measures by governments or even involving the military in otherwise social issues. Elbe (2010) discusses the negative effects of securitizing health threats on international cooperative efforts to address these with reference to Indonesia's refusal to share national viral samples with the rest of the international community in the context of the avian influenza (H5N1) epidemic. This decision was in response to concerns with vaccine supply and some governments' stockpiling of available vaccines, which left other governments unable to procure vaccines even though their populations were likely to need these more.

Elbe (2006) warns of the ethical dilemmas of linking HIV/AIDS and security – namely, the term security evoking threat-defence associations, prompting excessive state mobilization, or removing the issue from the realm of everyday politics and moving it into the realm of politics of exception, defined by strategic decision-making, which tends to be more urgent and less consultative, transparent or accountable. Nunes expresses concern with the dynamics of domination and power inequality embedded in security and health security politics, which may leave 'dominated groups vulnerable to decisions and outcomes with a high impact upon their lives, and which they cannot control or even predict' (2014: 946). These concerns align with the view from critical security studies that security is about ensuring that individuals are both able to survive and able to make choices and maintain some autonomy in shaping their own lives.

The development of a more nuanced understanding of the links between global health and security politics and of the implications of such understanding for both health and security, requires scholars and practitioners on both sides to engage in a more effective, critical and inclusive dialogue. Such dialogue requires an inter-disciplinary approach and the engagement of both theoretical and empirically-informed thinking as a way of gaining a systematic and in-depth understanding capable of incorporating broader conceptualizations of the relationship between security and health, as well as insights from practice. The global health community has an important role to play in this dialogue – drawing on its own practice, observations, lived experiences – to affect world affairs, social and political change.

Activity 8.2

Think of a global public health issue and consider the following questions: Are there advantages or disadvantages to health outcomes if the issue is framed as a threat to *national security*? Are health outcomes likely to change if the issue is framed as a *human security* issue? What positive or negative effects do you think the security community could identify in incorporating selected health problems into its agenda?

Feedback

In considering the above, you will need to think about what different goals and perspectives the health and security communities might have, as well as their different degrees of influence over the political agenda. The health community might benefit from the raising of selected health issues higher on the public policy agenda. However, this might be at the expense of skewing the agenda and thus neglecting other, equally pressing, health needs. The security community could benefit from dealing in a timely and appropriate manner with a real threat to a population's well-being. However, it may also be seen as risking the opening up of the security agenda too broadly.

Summary

This chapter offered a discussion of the links between health and security, grounded in a more detailed conceptual understanding of security debates in international relations. It presented competing and conflicting views, critical reasoning and perspectives on how security and health interact, how they *ought to* interact and what some of the implications of these interactions might be. There are benefits and drawbacks to conceptualizing health as a security concern. On the one hand, if health is framed as a national security issue, priority attention and resources are easier to mobilize; on the other hand, there are normative and practical concerns with the appropriateness of such framing. Health issues and their profound existential impacts on individuals and communities, however, can be used as a starting point to reconsider how we think about security and security politics. Health security politics can lead the way in conceptualizing security away from exceptional, antagonistic state-level politics and the mobilization of military resources, towards cooperative, empowering, human-centred, transnational efforts to protect human life.

References

Booth, K. (2007) *Theory of World Security*. Cambridge: Cambridge University Press.
Brainard, L. and Chollet, D. (eds) (2007) *Too Poor for Peace? Global Poverty, Conflict, and Security in the 21st Century*. Washington, DC: Brookings Institution Press.
Brown, G. and Stoeva, P. (2015) Reevaluating health security from a cosmopolitan perspective, in S. Rushton and J. Youde (eds) *Routledge Handbook of Global Health Security*. London: Routledge.

Buzan, B. (1991) *People, States and Fear: An Agenda for International Security Studies in the Post-Cold War Era*, 2nd edn. London: Harvester Wheatsheaf.

Collier, P. (2008) *The Bottom Billion: Why the Poorest Countries Are Failing and What Can Be Done About It*. Oxford: Oxford University Press.

Commission on Human Security (2003) *Human Security Now*. New York: Commission on Human Security.

Council of the European Union (2003) *A Secure Europe in a Better World*, Brussels, 12 December 2003. Available at: https://data.consilium.europa.eu/doc/document/ST-15895-2003-INIT/en/pdf (accessed 28 May 2021).

Dewachi, O., Skelton, M., Nguyen, V. et al. (2014) Changing therapeutic geographies of the Iraqi and Syrian Wars, *The Lancet*, 383(9915): 449–457.

Elbe, S. (2006) Should HIV/AIDS be securitized? The ethical dilemmas of linking HIV/AIDS and security, *International Studies Quarterly*, 50(1): 119–144.

Elbe, S. (2010) Haggling over viruses: the downside risks of securitizing infectious disease, *Health Policy and Planning*, 25: 476–485.

Feldbaum, H. and Lee, K. (2004) Public health and security, in A. Ingram (ed.) *Health, Foreign Policy and Security – Towards a Conceptual Framework for Research and Policy*. UK Global Health Programme Working Paper 2. London: The Nuffield Trust.

Fidler, D. (2003) Public health and national security in the global age: infectious diseases, bioterrorism and realpolitik, *George Washington International Law Review*, 35: 787–856.

Garrett, L. (1996) The return of infectious disease, *Foreign Affairs*, 75: 66–79.

Holst, J. (2020) Global health – emergence, hegemonic trends and biomedical reductionism, *Globalization and Health*, 16(1): 42.

Institute of Medicine (IOM) (1997) *America's Vital Interest in Global Health: Protecting Our People, Enhancing Our Economy, and Advancing Our International Interests*. Washington, DC: National Academies Press. Available at: http://globalization.nap.edu/openbook.php?record_id=5717 (accessed 28 May 2021).

McInnes, C. (2011) HIV, AIDS and conflict in Africa: why isn't it (even) worse, *Review of International Studies,* 37(2): 485–509.

McSweeney, B. (1999) *Security, Identity and Interests: A Sociology of International Relations*. Cambridge: Cambridge University Press.

Nunes, J. (2014) Questioning health security: insecurity and domination in world politics, *Review of International Studies*, 40(5): 939–960.

Peterson, S. (2002) Epidemic disease and national security, *Security Studies*, 12(2): 43–81.

Price-Smith, A. (2009) *Contagion and Chaos: Disease, Ecology, and National Security in the Era of Globalization*. Cambridge, MA: MIT Press.

Quinn, J., Stoeva, P., Zeleny, T. et al. (2017) Public health crisis: the need for primary prevention in failed and fragile states, *Central European Journal of Public Health*, 25(3): 171–176.

Rushton, S. (2011) Global health security: security for whom? Security from what?, *Political Studies*, 59(4): 779–796.

Shamasunder, S., Holmes, S., Goronga, T. et al. (2020) Covid-19 reveals weak health systems by design: why we must re-make global health in this historic moment, *Global Public Health*, 15(7): 1083–1089.

Stoddard, A., Harvey, P., Czwarno, M. et al. (2020) Aid worker security report 2020: contending with threats to humanitarian health workers in the age of epidemics. Humanitarian Outcomes. Available at: https://globalization.humanitarianoutcomes.org/AWSR2020 (accessed 28 May 2021).

United Nations Development Programme (1994) *Human Development Report 1994: New Dimensions of Human Security*. Oxford: Oxford University Press.

United Nations Human Security Unit (2016) *Human Security Handbook*. Available at: https://globalization.un.org/humansecurity/wp-content/uploads/2017/10/h2.pdf (accessed 28 May 2021).

US National Intelligence Council (2000) National intelligence estimate: the global infectious disease threat and its implications for the United States, *Environmental Change and Security Project Report*, 6: 33–65.

World Health Organization (WHO) (2020) The top 10 causes of death. Available at: https://globalization.who.int/news-room/fact-sheets/detail/the-top-10-causes-of-death (accessed 10 June 2021).

World Health Organization (WHO) (2021a) Noncommunicable diseases. Key facts. Available at: https://globalization.who.int/news-room/fact-sheets/detail/noncommunicable-diseases (accessed 28 May 2021).

World Health Organization (WHO) (2021b) [@WHO]. 2021, Feb, 23. 'I said that global health security is only as strong as its weakest link – no one is safe until we are all safe' – @DrTedros. Twitter. Available at: https://twitter.com/WHO/status/1364259167876362242 (accessed June 2021).

Williams, P. and McDonald M. (2018) An introduction to security studies, in P. Williams and M. McDonald (eds) *Security Studies: An Introduction*. London: Routledge.

PART 3

Global health governance

The state as an actor in global health

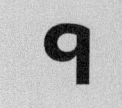

Benjamin Hawkins

Overview

This chapter examines the nature of the state as a political entity and the crucial importance of states as actors within global health governance. To understand the role of the state in global health requires an appreciation of how its status and functions differ between the domestic (i.e. national) and global (i.e. supra-national) spheres. In addition, this chapter will explore how the role of the state as an actor in global health has been affected by the emergence of important non-state actors, such as corporations and civil society organizations. It will assess the continued importance of the state as a global health actor, including the key role played by states within international organizations and other bilateral and multilateral entities within the institutional architecture of global health.

Learning objectives

After working through this chapter, you will be able to:

- Define the state as a political entity.
- Differentiate between the role of the state in domestic and global politics.
- Critically appraise the legacy of colonialism and enduring power asymmetries on the functioning of the state in different contexts.
- Contrast the nature and functions of the state with that of other key actors in global health policy.
- Evaluate the extent to which the state remains the predominant actor in global health.

Key terms

The state: A nation or territory that constitutes an organized political community under a government. The term is often used to denote the government of a particular territory, especially in the context of international organizations and the discipline of international relations, which analyses political interactions between states.

Domestic politics: This refers to policymaking and governance activities within the confines of the territorial state. It is sometimes referred to as national politics (as opposed to supra-national politics at the level above the state).

International relations: The conduct of policy above the level of the state and the discipline devoted to its study.

The idea of the state

Within the field of political philosophy, attempts to theorize the role of the state and the limits of state power extend back thousands of years. Plato's *Republic* (written around 375 BCE), for example, is an attempt to work out the ideal model for the state. The early Islamic philosopher and jurist, Al-Fabri, likewise sought to chart the parameters of the 'virtuous city' as an early form of the state (Kurmangaliyeva and Azerbayev 2016). These attempts continue up to the present day and are at the heart of some of the fiercest political and ideological debates. Some commentators emphasize the need for the state to protect citizens and provide public services which meet their needs. Others, meanwhile, are wary of what they see as the state stepping beyond its legitimate political remit and into areas of citizens' lives in which it (arguably) has no right to intervene.

This has implications for debates about the appropriate role of the state in the implementation of health policy and the provision and financing of health services. For example, issues such the regulation of harmful products like tobacco, alcohol and processed food turn on whether the state should be able to control what individuals consume, even where this may be motivated by a desire to protect their health. This becomes an even more complex question when we consider that the behaviours of some individuals (e.g. those who smoke) may impose harms on others and costs on the health system, which are paid for by other citizens (i.e. through taxation or higher insurance premiums), or may divert limited resources away from treating other conditions and diseases or other area of public policy (e.g. education or transportation).

✏ **Activity 9.1**

Drawing on what you have learned in previous chapters, and your own experience, list the three to four key roles of the state as a political actor in the field of national and global health governance. When you have done this, try to come up with a definition of the state in one or two sentences. Does your definition cover the role of the state at both the national and global level, or do these require separate definitions? How does its role differ between these contexts? Compare your definition with the discussion of the state in each context below.

Within the social sciences, a distinction is drawn in the role of the state between the domestic (national) and the global (supra-national) spheres. The so-called 'internal' and 'external' functions of the state are the objects of study of the disciplines of *political science* and *international relations* (IR), respectively. These disciplines make very different assumptions about the nature of the state and its ability to govern effectively in the policy contexts on which they principally focus.

The state and domestic politics

Numerous attempts have been made to define, describe, justify and critique the role of the state within the domestic sphere. Thomas Hobbes (1960 [1651]) argued that the state is necessary to regulate the interactions between individuals; to create an overarching authority that can regulate their behaviour and enforce laws. The role of the state is, therefore, to govern social relations to the overall benefit of the citizenry, to act as an arbiter between citizens, to manage conflict and enforce social order. While the necessity of the state is widely accepted by almost all political theorists, significant disagreement exists about the degree to which it ought to intervene in citizens' affairs and seek to shape society. This has obvious implications for the right of the state to levy taxes and to redistribute wealth through the tax system and, as such, is at the heart of contemporary debates about the funding of the welfare state in many countries and also the legitimacy of taxation being used to fund overseas aid and development spending.

Perhaps the most famous and often quoted definition of the role of the state is that it is 'a monopoly over the legitimate use of violence' (Weber 1972 [1919]). That is to say, the state – in the domestic sphere – has the right to employ physical coercion in order to enforce the rule of law and that its ability to do so is both legally inscribed and accepted by those it governs. In concrete terms, this means that the state may use a variety of means to get citizens to comply with the law, such as fining them or forbidding them to enter certain places, arresting them, placing them in jail or using electronic tagging devices to track their movements. However, this definition must be treated with care as there must be limits to the actions that states may justifiably take and the ends to which they can be used. It assumes the legitimacy of the state institutions is accepted by those governed and the use of coercion is limited to the enforcement of shared political objectives and norms. For example, governments may use arguments about public order, the need to enforce national law and to maintain security as a pretext for political repression of their citizens or of certain sub-populations.

Political scientists attempt to explain how the state functions and what the consequences of the state's activities are. This can be addressed from a range of perspectives, which make different assumptions about the neutrality of the state as a political entity and which emphasize different consequences of state behaviours for specific groups and sub-populations (Dryzek and Dunelavy 2009). Pluralist accounts of the state identify a multiplicity of relevant policy actors (e.g. individual citizens, collectives, trade unions, non-governmental and civil society organizations, businesses) competing for power and influence in different parts of the state apparatus and the machinery of government (see Dahl 1961). Marxist analyses, meanwhile, argue that the structures of the state serve the interests of those who control capital at the expense of the majority of the citizenry (see Milliband 1969). Feminist theories meanwhile emphasize the gendered nature of the state and the consequent marginalization of women and their political interests within the modern state (MacKinnon 1989). Post-colonial theorists meanwhile have identified how the specific experience of state formation in post-colonial societies has affected the structure and power relations within such states (see Amin-Khan 2013). An emerging literature is also increasingly focusing on the enduring effects of the experience of colonialism on imperial states such as the UK (see Sanghera 2021).

These approaches help us to understand the different ways in which resources are allocated within a given society, including the provision of health services and the design of health policies. Why is it that certain health issues and conditions are given greater priority than others? Why is it that certain groups are prioritized or marginalized within the health system or have better or worse health outcomes than others? Why are health policies and services organized and delivered in the way that they are? Understanding the structure and function of the state is crucial to being able to answer these fundamental questions.

It should be noted too that states differ in form. They may be unitary (i.e. governed as a single policy space), devolved (i.e. with responsibility for areas of policy or public administration passed to sub-national entities such as regions or cities) or federal (i.e. a more clearly defined and constitutionally delineated separation between the responsibilities of national/federal government and the constituent entities which form it). In both devolved and federal states, some decisions are taken, and policies made, at the national level and some are taken at a sub-national level of government, particularly in federal systems. Health policy is often devolved to sub-national entities or competence for it may be shared across levels of government. This can lead to greater local responsiveness, for example in heath service care provision, but also create issues for coordinated national responses to certain health issues and public health crises. It should be noted also that states may have different political characteristics, being democratic, partially democratic, autocratic or authoritarian in nature with implications for the organization and control of state institutions and the ability to enforce policy decisions, including the degree of control exercised by national government over sub-national entities. These factors will also impact health policy in various ways.

In the domestic sphere, the state has the capacity to confer certain health-based rights (e.g. access to healthcare), to place associated obligations on citizens (e.g. to pay taxes to fund health services) and to enforce adherence to relevant laws (e.g. restrictions on movement to prevent infectious disease outbreak) through potentially robust measures (i.e. fines and imprisonment). However, it should be acknowledged that the capacity of states to do this, in terms of available resources and infrastructure, varies greatly. In many contexts, such as conflict and post-conflict societies, the state may not be able to exercise effective control over all aspects of its territory or the degree of control may vary between regions (see Holden 2017). In others, the legitimate sovereignty of the state over some territorial spaces, and the right of state institutions to exercise control over this, may also be contested due to competing claims of different groups over specific territories.

The relevance of this discussion of the powers of the state for public health came to the fore once again (see Chapter 4 for earlier examples) during the Covid-19 pandemic when some states implemented extensive restrictions on the ability of citizens to exercise their fundamental rights and freedoms (e.g. their freedom of movement or association with others). This led to debates about whether such measures, and the penalties such as fines or even imprisonment for non-compliance, were justifiable to ensure the collective well-being and safety of the population. While the *de facto* ability of states to provide services, collect taxes and enforce health regulation may vary across the globe and is dependent on the resources and infrastructure to facilitate this, in principle at least these forms of revenue generation, enforcement (and coercion) remain open to states at the national level in ways which they are not at the supra-national or global level.

The state in the international sphere

While the activities of the state are vital in the implementation of global health policy, it is the role of the state at the supra-national level that is perhaps of most obvious relevance to the study of global health and global health governance. The function of the state in the global sphere differs greatly from that within the domestic sphere and is the focus of the discipline of IR (see Chapter 4). There are long-standing debates within IR about the function of the state and the capacity for collective political action at the global level. Despite wide differences in emphasis between theoretical approaches, there is a general consensus among scholars that states are concerned primarily with their own security and survival and, as a result of this, act in ways designed to secure their own interests (see McGlinchey et al. 2017). However, the extent to which states can achieve this varies enormously depending on economic, strategic and military capacity (see Chapter 8).

The key assumption in IR is that the global sphere is characterized by a state of *anarchy*. Anarchy, in this context, refers to the absence of an over-arching global authority to govern the relationship between states (i.e. a global government). In other words, there is no body at the global level which is able to play the equivalent role of the state in the domestic sphere by managing relations between states and enforcing international law. It is this condition that shapes state behaviour in the global sphere. While at the national level the state functions as an ultimate authority ensuring that individuals, and entities such as companies, non-governmental organiza-tions (NGOs), trade unions, etc., fulfil their obligations to one another, within the global system states must manage their relations with other states (and non-state actors) without recourse to an external authority or enforcement mechanism. Thus, there is an incentive for states to create mechanisms, structures and more formal institutions and organizations to regulate their interactions with other states and non-state actors and manage the effects of state behaviour.

These institutions can be seen as the means through which states have attempted to respond to the undermining of their capacity for effective unilateral action (e.g. on issues such as climate change) and the increas-ing interdependence between states brought about by these processes. Examples of such organizations include the United Nations (UN), the World Trade Organization (WTO), the World Health Organization (WHO), the World Bank and its sister organization the International Monetary Fund (IMF), the Organization for Economic Cooperation and Development (OECD), the G7 (formerly the G8), the G20, G77, G90 and the European Union (EU). Inter-national organizations are discussed in greater detail in Chapter 10. Here, it is sufficient to note the fact that these bodies are constituted by their member states and serve as a mechanism through which they seek to achieve their political objectives and protect their interests.

The role played by states within such organizations is central to under-standing the ongoing importance of the state as an actor in global health policy. However, there are limits to their effectiveness and their ability to govern state behaviour in the international sphere. States often do not adhere to the rules they agree to in forming or acceding to such bodies and international organizations often lack the ability to enforce these obligations on recalcitrant states. Moreover, there are huge variations in the ability of individual states to influence the activities of these structures. International organizations are often criticized for reflecting the power and interests of the biggest and wealthiest states, which provide much of their funding (see Chapter 10). As such, it may be particularly difficult to hold these powerful states to account. 'Critical' international relations theorists have identified the way in which these global institutions – particularly global economic institutions – established by the most powerful, high-income states, create structural dependencies between the 'Global North' and the 'Global South', or between what is termed 'core' states that set the rules of the game and the 'periphery' that depends on these states for their trade and security (see Wallerstein 1992).

These issues about the possibility for global cooperation and coordination between states and about non-compliance are of vital importance to debates in global health policy. For example, does the World Health Organization (WHO) have the right to demand countries disclose the details of outbreaks of contagious diseases in their territory in order to facilitate the development of vaccines and to prevent the spread of the pandemic? Does it have the ability to hold its most powerful member states to account for their non-compliance? Or is it the right of state governments to manage the crisis themselves?

The role of WHO and the International Health Regulations (IHR) in managing global infectious disease outbreaks highlights the competing priorities of states and the tensions which can exist between their internal (domestic) and external (global) responsibilities. The 2003 SARS outbreak and the political responses to this provides an important case study of these issues which has been the subject of significant attention by IR scholars and international global health lawyers. David Fidler (2004) argues that the 2003 outbreak marked a transition from a state-centred system based on the sovereignty of states over the treatment of disease outbreaks within their own territory to a system in which the international community, and the international organizations through which it acts, began to play a more robust role in the governance of these issues, intervening in the internal affairs of states in the name of the common welfare of the international community. According to Fidler, the emerging international system is marked by the 'decentring' of the role of the state and the increasing prominence of other, non-state actors. In contrast to Fidler's analysis, James Ricci (2009) argues that the global health governance literature has overstated the extent to which the role of the state in global health governance has diminished or been usurped by other actors, and cites evidence of the continued importance of the state in global health governance. The SARS case provides important context for the issues raised by current events in global health. Parallels to this case are found in the political responses to the 2014 West African Ebola outbreak (Moon et al. 2015) and, most recently, Covid-19 pandemic since 2019 (IPPPR 2021). Criticism of the global health response to the Ebola crisis centred on many of the same issues raised by SARS. While detailed, scholarly analyses of the political response to the Covid-19 pandemic are largely still to be written, and the situation continues to evolve, questions have already arisen about the role played by WHO in managing a crisis of such obvious global significance, including whether the international alert mechanisms for disease outbreaks such as that which occurred in Wuhan, China, in December 2019 are fit for purpose, and whether adequate resources are in place to oversee these (IPPPR 2021). Tensions have also emerged within WHO, and the wider international community, about the global handling of the pandemic in ways which highlight the reliance on international systems on the engagement and compliance of states (IPPPR 2021).

✎ Activity 9.2

Think about an international organization of which your home country is a member. What are the reasons why states would adhere to the rules this organization establishes? Why may they break these rules? What consequences would your country experience if it did break these rules? How would the organization/other member states respond to this?

Feedback

A potentially helpful way to think about this is in terms of incentives and costs. There may be strong incentives for a state to try to 'game' the system or to interpret rules in ways which favour its interests over those of other states and thereby gain an advantage over them. And limited costs for non-compliance due to the weak enforcement mechanisms available. In the WTO, for example, which limits the subsidies that member state governments can give to domestic industries in order to ensure 'fair' competition between businesses across the globe, it may be advantageous for states to support businesses that are a source of taxation and employment. Enforcement in the WTO is via retaliatory measures from other states following a long dispute resolution process. These include adding tariffs to imported goods from the offending state to make these more expensive and thus undesirable in their market. However, this may not be a deterrent for states such as the US or blocs such as the EU, which, as large economies, are far less dependent on trade with smaller complainant states and may be prepared to accept retaliatory measures as the price for subsidizing key strategic industries. At the same time, states may seek to avoid costs which are imposed on them by international organizations, for example by refusing to pay designated budgetary contributions, as is the case with the US and WHO. This refusal to pay for the costs of an organization while enjoying the benefits is known in economics as the 'free rider' problem. In the example above, it may be the case that states subject to an

infectious disease outbreak are worried about the political and reputa-
tional damage that may arise from being seen to be the source of a new
pandemic, or having failed to act appropriately to control it. This may
affect perceptions of that state as a trustworthy partner for other states
or for businesses seeking to invest there. It may deter tourism and
travel. As such there are incentives for seeking to underplay or manage
perceptions of such an outbreak. As we have seen though, these actions
can lead to a worsening of the situation on the ground and ultimately to
greater political and economic damage in addition to greater mortality
and morbidity from the disease.

The state, globalization and health

Processes of globalization have led to the emergence of new types of
global policy and regulatory issues that require global solutions. For example, the health challenges posed by the large-scale movement of people
across the globe may facilitate or accelerate the spread of infectious diseases (see Chapter 5) and may be a factor in environmental degradation
which is a key structural determinant of health (see Chapter 7). Similarly,
changes in the structure of the global economy (Chapter 2) have led to an
erosion of the power of states to regulate transnational economic activity
and global corporations involved in the sale and marketing of health-
harming products such as tobacco, alcohol and processed food whose
economic resources outstrip those of many states (see Chapter 11). The
inability of states to act unilaterally to police the activities of corporations,
for example, undermines their *de facto* control, or sovereignty, over certain
policy issues. Perhaps as a consequence of this, recent decades have
witnessed the emergence of a myriad of non-state actors in the field of
global health, including NGOs, charitable organizations, policy networks
that have sought to fill the regulatory gaps between states and new governance structures and mechanisms for policy delivery that offer greater
prominence to non-state actors than is the case in traditional international
organizations (see Chapter 12).

Box 9.1   Case study: The Framework Convention on Tobacco Control

The Framework Convention on Tobacco Control (FCTC) was WHO's first
attempt to exercise its constitutional authority to develop a global public
health treaty. The final text of the agreement was drafted by an Inter-
governmental Negotiating Body (INB) and unanimously endorsed by the
56th World Health Assembly in May 2003. Based on recognition of the

challenges posed by globalization, the FCTC is intended to address transnational issues and provide a powerful resource to support national health efforts. The FCTC includes a series of 'best practices' in tobacco control policy setting out a blueprint for national governments to follow in supporting population health and reducing smoking rates. Moreover, the FCTC provided an important reference point for public health and tobacco control.

Article 5.3 of the FCTC aims to restrict the influence of the tobacco industry over policymaking. The FCTC also creates the mechanism for the development of subsequent protocols on specific areas of tobacco control issues of international concerns (e.g. tobacco smuggling and illicit trade which was the focus of the first such protocol). However, progress on developing these protocols has been slow. This reflects the enormous complexity of drafting regulations that suit such a wide array of countries and their differing political priorities and for the protocol to be signed and subsequently ratified by national governments and legislatures before entering into force. Reporting on FCTC implementation suggests also that this has been piecemeal (Fooks et al. 2017).

The FCTC was vehemently opposed by cigarette producers who saw it as 'an unprecedented challenge to the tobacco industry's freedom to continue doing business' (BAT Indonesia n.d.). They sought to build support among potentially sympathetic states and ministers who may be willing to oppose the agreement or able to influence its content and sought to place their representatives within national negotiating delegations.

The FCTC process also entailed efforts to include civil society under the auspices of the Framework Convention Alliance (FCA). This proved to be a source of tension within a fundamentally state-centric policy process and the terms of participation of NGOs remained strongly contested throughout the negotiation process. The impact of civil society in the final negotiations was significantly hampered by increasing unease among member states opposed to the agreement of such a powerful text and NGO actors saw a reduction of access and transparency in the final meetings of the INB, which was reportedly supported by delegations including the USA and China.

The case of the FCTC demonstrates again the crucial role of state actors as key decision-makers. They are the principal agents in international organizations such as WHO and able to enact measures such as the framework and its protocols. They too are largely responsible for its implementations. Yet state actions occur in a context in which other actors are also influential. NGOs advocate for health protective measures and hold governments to account while powerful transnational companies may lobby state delegations to oppose these.

The continuing relevance of the state

In this context, questions arise over the relative importance of the state as an actor in the field of global health compared to civil society and commercial actors, and whether the state remains the pre-eminent policy actor in the global sphere? While the hegemony of the state as a global health actor has been 'decentred' by processes of globalization, it remains a key global health actor for a number of reasons.

First, much global health financing continues to be provided by states. For example, over 90 per cent of the Global Fund 'recharges' as well as the majority of WHO budget contributions come from states (World Economic Forum 2020).

Second, states remain the dominant political actors within the key structures and institutions through which global health governance occurs (such as the UN or WHO). Decision-making within these organizations and the principal policy initiatives that emerge from them, such as the Sustainable Development Goals (SDGs), reflect the priorities and constraints placed on global health action of their member states, albeit in collaboration with other actors. While international organizations may establish forums for civil society or commercial actors and create mechanisms through which they can feed into policy discussions – for example, the recognition of 'social partners' at the UN High Level Meetings on NCDs – their status is fundamentally different from that of the member states. At the WTO, for example, it is only states that have the capacity to initiate disputes against other member states for alleged violations of trade law and private citizens and companies have no legal standing.

Third, the implementation of global health policy initiatives on the ground depend on state structures and support. For example, global vaccination initiatives will depend in part on local structures and actors to deliver these, while the Paris Agreement, within the UN Framework Convention on Climate Change, depends on states acting at the domestic level to deliver on commitments. The continuing importance of the states, and their interactions with other global health actors, is evident in the examples of the WHO Framework Convention on Tobacco Control (FCTC; Box 9.1) and the provision of medication to tackle the HIV/Aids pandemic (Box 9.2).

It should be highlighted though that the continued importance of the state in global health, as discussed so far, underplays the significant variations in power and capacity which exist between states. The ability of economically and politically less powerful states to shape global health policy will be far more limited than larger, richer states that exert significant influence over these forums. The interests of low- and middle-income countries (LMICs) may often be more effectively represented through collective action (e.g. via the G77 or G90 group of the world's poorest states, which has sought to influence WTO negotiations) or via the activities of influential civil society actors with political traction in high-income settings. Similarly, these states will often be net recipients of financing from, rather than funders of, global health programmes. In keeping with this, they will be more dependent on outside support from donor organizations to implement global health initiatives on the ground.

Box 9.2   Case study: The state and the fight against HIV/ AIDS

The crucial issue in the fight against HIV/AIDS centres on access to (expensive) anti-retroviral medications, or ARVs, by those infected by HIV in LMICs where the majority of the world's known cases of HIV infection are found. Access to these medicines is restricted by the enormous cost of patented drugs and the inability to produce cheaper generic versions of ARVs due to the protection of drug companies' intellectual property rights under international patent law and WTO agreements including the Agreement on Trade Related Aspects of Intellectual Property (TRIPs). Thus, there is a potential conflict between the intellectual property rights of drug companies on the one hand and the need for drugs by those in the LMICs on the other. This was evident in 2001 when the government of South Africa adopted measures to allow 'parallel import' of generic ARVs and issued compulsory licences for their domestic manufacture – thereby undercutting the price of branded medicines – in order to tackle the health crisis it was facing. For further details on the background to the WTO system and the TRIPs agreement in this case see Chapter 13.

State actors have played a crucial role in these developments. It was state actors who concluded the Uruguay Round of negotiations that brought the WTO into being, along with the agreement, TRIPS, which is designed to protect intellectual property rights. In particular, the US government was vital in negotiating the TRIPS agreement at the WTO and insisted on the inclusion of protection for pharmaceuticals in it (Sell 2003).

Civil society organizations (CSOs) such as Médecins Sans Frontière and the Red Cross have played a crucial role in bringing the issue of HIV and ARV provision onto the global policy agenda and are intimately involved in the treatment of patients and the distribution of medication in many countries (see Chapter 11). Yet much of their activity remains dependent on the role of states to facilitate their work.

States also provide the 'hardware' of public healthcare (Fidler 2007). They often produce the overall strategies for tackling health issues like HIV/AIDS and state agencies play a central role in implementing these strategies and delivering screening and treatment on the ground

(Wogart et al. 2009). The governments of high-income countries provide overseas aid that is used to tackle issues such as HIV/AIDS through agencies such USAID, the US International Development Agency, or the Foreign Commonwealth and Development Office (FCDO) in the UK.

There are various supranational bodies and international organizations active in the field of HIV/AIDS, including the World Bank Multi-country AIDS Projects, the G7, the Office of the United Nations High Commissioner for Refugees (UNHCR) and UNAIDS. However, it is crucial to remember that states play a vital role in the governance and funding of these bodies. In addition, global health partnerships, most notably the Global Fund, involve a variety of different agencies and civil society actors working together in the fight against AIDS (see Chapter 12). It should be noted though that states provide the overwhelming majority of funding channelled through the Global Fund. The process of tackling HIV/AIDS involves a complex interplay of state and non-state actors and it is difficult to assess the relative contribution made by these actors, but it is undeniable that the state continues to play a central role in the fight against HIV/AIDS.

✎ Activity 9.3

Think about the areas of global health governance we have looked at. In which areas has the state played the most important role? In which areas has its role been usurped by other actors? Which actors were these and why did they assume the role they did? Summarize your findings in a brief paragraph giving examples to support your points.

Re-read the definition of the state you wrote at the start of the chapter. Reflect on whether your understanding of the state has changed and, if so, how. If your understanding has changed, write a new definition of the role of the state that reflects your current understanding.

Summary

In summary, this chapter identified how there are important differences between the role of the state at the domestic and global levels and that the function of the state as a global health actor differs in each context. It highlighted also the very different capacity of states to influence global health and global health governance, related to their political and economic power and their experience of colonialism. Moreover, processes of globalization have posed new challenges to the state in the health arena. There is an increasing number of non-state actors, for example global corporations (see Chapter 11) and international non-governmental organizations (see Chapter 12) that are of importance in different areas of global health governance. Nevertheless, states remain arguably the most important of all of these actors, playing a vital role in the design, funding and implementation of global health policy.

References

Amin-Khan, T. (2013) *The Post-Colonial State in the Era of Capitalist Globalization: Historical, Political and Theoretical Approaches to State Formation*. London: Routledge.

BAT Indonesia (n.d.) *A Study on the Smokers of International Brands*. Guildford Depository, Bates No. 400458935–9056.

Dahl, R.A. (1961) *Who Governs? Power and Democracy in an American City*. New Haven, CT: Yale University Press.

Dryzek, J. and Dunleavy, P. (2009) *Theories of the Democratic State*. London: Macmillan International Higher Education.

Fidler, D.P. (2004) *SARS: Governance and the Globalization of Disease*. London: Palgrave Macmillan.

Fidler, D. (2007) Architecture amidst anarchy: global health's quest for governance, *Global Health Governance*, 1(1): 1–17.

Fooks, G.J., Smith, J., Lee, K. et al. (2017) Controlling corporate influence in health policy making? An assessment of the implementation of article 5.3 of the World Health Organization framework convention on tobacco control, *Globalization and Health*, 13(1): 1–20.

Hobbes, T. (1960 [1651]) *Leviathan: Or the Matter, Forme and Power of a Commonwealth Ecclesiasticall and Civil*. New Haven, CT: Yale University Press.

Holden, C. (2017) Graduated sovereignty and global governance gaps: special economic zones and the illicit trade in tobacco products, *Political Geography*, 59: 72–81.

Independent Panel on Pandemic Preparedness and Response (IPPPR) (2021) *Second Report on Progress*. Prepared for the WHO executive Broad. Available at: https://theindependentpanel.org/wp-content/uploads/2021/01/Independent-Panel_Second-Report-on-Progress_Final-15-Jan-2021.pdf (accessed 8 November 2021).

Kurmangaliyeva, G. and Azerbayev, A. (2016) Al-Farabi's virtuous city and its contemporary significance, *The Anthropologist*, 26(1): 88–96.

MacKinnon, C. (1989) *Toward a Feminist Theory of the State*. Cambridge, MA: Harvard University Press.

McGlinchey, S., Walters, R. and Scheinpflug, C. (2017) *International Relations Theory*. Bristol: E-International Relations. Available at: http://globalization.e-ir.info/wp-content/uploads/2017/11/International-Relations-Theory-E-IR.pdf (accessed 8 November 2021).

Miliband, R. (1969) *The State in Capitalist Society*. London: Weidenfeld & Nicolson.

Moon, S., Sridhar, D., Pate, M. et al. (2015) Will Ebola change the game? Ten essential reforms before the next pandemic. The report of the Harvard-LSHTM Independent Panel on the Global Response to Ebola, *Lancet*, 386(10009): 2204–2221.

Ricci, J. (2009) Global health governance and the state: premature claims of a post-international framework, *Global Health*, 3(1): 1–18.

Sanghera, S. (2021) *Empireland*. London: Penguin.

Sell, S.K. (2003) *Private Power, Public Law: The Globalization of Intellectual Property Rights*. Cambridge: Cambridge University Press.

Wallerstein, I. (1992) The West, capitalism, and the modern world-system, *Review (Fernand Braudel Center)*, 15(4): 561–619.

Waxman, H.A. (2004) Politics of international health in the Bush Administration, *Development*, 47(2): 24–28.

Weber, M. (1972 [1919]) *Politics as a Vocation*. Philadelphia, PA: Fortress Press.

Wogart, J.P., Calcagnotto, G., Hein, W. et al. (2009) AIDS and access to medicines: Brazil, South Africa and global health governance, in K. Buse, W. Hein and N. Drager (eds) *Making Sense of Global Health Governance: A Policy Perspective*. Basingstoke: Palgrave Macmillan.

World Economic Forum (2020) *How Is the World Health Organization Funded?* Available at: https://globalization.weforum.org/agenda/2020/04/who-funds-world-health-organization-un-coronavirus-pandemic-covid-trump/ (accessed 8 November 2021).

10 Bilateral, multilateral and regional actors in global health

Benjamin Hawkins and Marco Liverani

Overview

Building on the previous chapter on the role of the state in health governance, this chapter focuses on the bilateral and multilateral agreements, alliances and institutional structures formed by states to cooperate and manage public health issues of international concern. Multilateral cooperation arrangements are discussed both at the global and regional level. At the global level, this chapter discusses the United Nations (UN) system and the various agencies within this as they relate to health, including the World Health Organization (WHO). In addition, it discusses global economic organizations such as the World Trade Organization (WTO), the World Bank (WB) and the International Monetary Fund (IMF), which have key impacts on economy development and thus health. The analysis of regional bodies focuses on the European Union (EU), the most developed example of regional political and economic integration, and compares and contrasts this to similar entities elsewhere in the world. The themes discussed in this chapter relate to other chapters in Part 2 including Chapter 9 on the state as a global health actor, Chapter 11 on the commercial sector and Chapter 12 on non-governmental actors in global health.

Learning objectives

After working through this chapter, you will be able to:

- Distinguish between bilateral, multilateral, global and regional forms of cooperation in the context of globalization.
- Analyse the way in which these different types of organizations, structures and cooperative arrangements impact on global health.
- Critically assess the role of the state and other global health actors in each type of entity as they relate to global health policy.

Key terms

Bilateral cooperation: The relationship, both formal and informal, between two states. This may be in the forms of officially codified and legally enforceable trade agreements or looser forms of engagement.

> **Multilateral cooperation:** Relationships formed between multiple actors, often enshrined in international organizations such as the United Nations and UN agencies, including the WHO and the World Trade Organization (WTO).
>
> **Intergovernmental organization:** A political entity above the supranational level, formed and governed by member states in dialogue with other entities such as civil society actors. These may be global (e.g. the United Nations or WTO) or regional (e.g. the EU or African Union) in nature.

Bilateral agreements

Bilateral agreements are those concluded between two parties, which may be two states or a state and a civil society entity. Bilateral agreements are often associated with the financing of particular health programmes in low- and middle-income countries (LMICs). For example, the President's Emergency Plan for AIDS Relief (PEPFAR) was established in 2003 by the US government to fund a range of HIV-related programmes in low-income countries (USDS 2021). Since then, PEPFAR has supported HIV treatment, prevention and care for millions of people through bilaterally-funded programmes in more than 85 countries. However, critics have argued that bilateral programmes serve as a means through which donors can exercise direct control over how their funds are allocated and applied, and also allow funders to promote particular forms of intervention that are in keeping with the underlying ideology of the funder. Elements of the programmes funded by PEPFAR under President George Bush were criticized on precisely these grounds (Evertz 2010).

Bilateral agreements in the field of international trade may also have important global health implications. As the Doha Round of WTO negotiations stalled in the early 2000s (see Chapter 13), states began to negotiate an increasing number of bilateral (and inter-regional) trade agreements with one another. These agreements have particular consequences for global health, prioritizing trade over health, providing corporations with extensive powers to challenge domestic policies under so-called 'investor state dispute settlement' (ISDS) mechanisms. For example, the global cigarette manufacturer Philip Morris has used these mechanisms to challenge tobacco control policies in Uruguay and Australia (Jarman 2015) (see Chapter 13).

It is important to note that there is often an asymmetry of power between the parties to a bilateral agreement, which usually reflects the size of the countries involved in terms of population and economic strength. Most obviously this is evident in the relations between donor and recipient countries, which are frequently discussed in the area of global health. However, in other settings agreements are often negotiated in a way that reflects the relative resources of the participants. This is a key difficulty for smaller states negotiating with larger partners and demonstrates how and why plurilateral and multilateral negotiations can be advantageous for such countries who may be able to form alliances, negotiate as a bloc or play off the interests of one larger partner against those of another. However, even in multilateral settings, power relations shape the content of the agreement and the interests of smaller states are often side-lined by the larger, more powerful countries and regions.

Activity 10.1

Identify a bilateral agreement between your country and another country. What is the purpose or the main objectives of this agreement? What rights and responsibilities does it create for the signatory states? What are its potential public health implications? Are these explicitly recognized or addressed in the agreement? Have any scholars or civil society organizations written about this agreement's effects on health?

Feedback

As we have seen above, there are multiple ways in which bilateral agreements, particularly trade and investment agreements, can affect health. For example, they may facilitate the importation of health products and equipment or the movement of healthcare providers and patients, but they may also facilitate the importation of food with differing standards or allow overseas companies to provide health services. In addition, they may include regulatory cooperation or dispute resolution mechanisms through which domestic laws can be challenged by other states or even by private actors such as corporations. However, such agreements often recognize the need to protect public health and include explicitly public health exceptions or justifications to divert from the terms of the agreement in certain circumstances.

Intergovernmental organizations as a response to globalization

Intergovernmental organizations (IGOs) are institutions that bring together three or more states to work together on issues that are relevant to all of them. As such, they are often called multilateral organizations to distinguish them from bilateral organizations involving only two parties. Examples of such organizations include the United Nations, the World Trade Organization (WTO), the World Health Organization (WHO), the World Bank (WB) and its sister organization the International Monetary Fund (IMF), the Organization for Economic Cooperation and Development (OECD), regional organizations such as the EU and the African Union, and looser associations of states with shared or common interests such as the G7, the G20, G77 and G90.

The development of intergovernmental organizations reflects increasing global interdependence and can be seen as a means through which states have attempted to respond to the undermining of their capacity for effective unilateral action. Thus, a central question in international relations (IR) that is of great importance for our understanding of global health, is to what extent IGOs enhance or undermine the power of the state. On the one hand, states retain a strong input into the decision-making structures of IGOs. Whereas other organizations may be officially recognized by IGOs or may have observer status, states are full members and are at the heart of the decision-making processes of these organizations. On the other hand, however, not all states have equal political input into these decision-making processes. So some states may retain a high level of control over policies decided within an IGO, while smaller, poorer states may have little *de facto* input. In addition, states do not retain complete control over the organizations they create. The secretariat and officials of intergovernmental organizations may be able to exert considerable influence over the direction and content of the measures adopted within their institutions. The extent to which states retain control varies between institutions. While most intergovernmental organizations remain overwhelmingly inter-governmental in nature – depending on the member states for their ultimate authority and guided in the substance of their position by the most powerful members – other IGOs such as the European Union (EU) have a more robust and influential supranational component in the form of the European Commission. The Commission exercises considerable influence over EU legislation through its right to propose and draft laws that are ratified by the European Parliament and the member states in the body known as the Council. In the following sections, we will discuss these issues and their global health implications in relation to the UN system and regional organizations such as the EU and the African Union.

The UN system and the World Health Organization

The UN is a large multipurpose international organization, representing nearly all the world's sovereign states. It was established after the end of the Second World War to prevent future conflicts, succeeding the ineffective League of Nations. In addition to maintaining international peace and security, the UN aims to protect human rights, to deliver humanitarian aid, to promote sustainable development and to uphold international law. It also serves as a forum where member countries can discuss and coordinate their actions to achieve these aims. Its aims and remit are set out in the 1945 United Nations Charter, which is an international legal document placing binding obligations on signatory states (Hanhimäki 2015).

The UN has six main bodies: the General Assembly, the Security Council, the Economic and Social Council (ECOSOC), the Trusteeship Council, the International Court of Justice and the Secretariat. The General Assembly is the main deliberative organ of the UN, where each member state has one vote regardless of its size or influence. The primary role of the General Assembly is to discuss issues and to make recommendations or 'resolutions', though it has no power to enforce them or compel state action. Furthermore, there is a multitude of specialized UN agencies and related bodies. These agencies are largely independent from the UN General Assembly and Secretary-General, with their own budgets and executive boards. Major specialized agencies include the International Labour Organization (ILO), the Food and Agriculture Organization (FAO), the United Nations Educational, Scientific and Cultural Organization (UNESCO), the United Nations Children Fund (UNICEF), the United Nations Development Programme (UNDP), the United Nations Environment Programme (UNEP), UN-Habitat and the World Health Organization (WHO). The World Bank and the International Monetary Fund (IMF) are two of the most powerful UN agencies and are also the most independent with respect to UN decision-making. The UN and its specialized agencies are often referred to collectively as the United Nations system.

In the past decades, the UN has expanded its operations to undertake a wide range of global development activities, including the design and implementation of major initiatives such as the Millennium Development Goals (MDGs) and the Sustainable Development Goals (SDGs). Derived from the Millennium Declaration, which was signed by 189 countries in September 2000, the MDGs (2000–2015) aimed to tackle some of the most pressing global issues including poverty, illiteracy and ill-health. The MDGs gained wide political support and shaped the global health agenda in the early 2000s, with their focus on reducing child mortality, improving maternal health and combating HIV/AIDS, malaria and other diseases (Marten 2018). In September 2015, the UN General Assembly adopted the SDGs (2015–2030), which replaced the MDGs by merging the agendas of development and environment. In the SDGs, the health-related goals were further expanded to 'ensure healthy lives and promote wellbeing for all at all ages', covering also the prevention and treatment of non-communicable diseases, substance abuse and road accidents.

The World Health Organization (WHO)

The WHO is the specialized health agency of the United Nations. As we discussed in Chapters 4 and 5, it was created in 1948 in the context of post-war initiatives to strengthen multilateral cooperation, replacing the Health Organization of the League of Nations in Geneva and the Office International d'Hygiène Publique (International Office of Public Health;

OIHP) in Paris (Cueto et al. 2019). As stated in its Constitution, the WHO was founded on the principles that 'the enjoyment of the highest attainable standard of health is one of the fundamental rights of every human being without distinction of race, religion, political belief, economic or social condition' and that 'the health of all peoples is fundamental to the attainment of peace and security and is dependent upon the fullest co-operation of individuals and States' (WHO 1948). Over the years this commitment to the universal right to health has been reasserted in various policy statements and campaigns including the Declaration of Alma-Ata and the Health for All movement in the 1970s (WHO 1978) and, more recently, the promotion of Universal Health Coverage, defined by the former WHO director-general Margaret Chanas 'the single most powerful concept that public health has to offer' (Chan 2012).

With administrative headquarters in Geneva, the WHO operates through the World Health Assembly, its supreme governance body, and through an Executive Board of health specialists, who implement the decisions and policy of the Health Assembly. The WHO Secretariat, which carries out routine operations and helps implement strategies, consists of experts and administrators based in Geneva or at one of the six regional offices or country offices around the world. The agency is led by a director general nominated by the Executive Board and appointed by the World Health Assembly. In 2017 Dr Tedros Adhanom Ghebreyesus became the first African to be appointed director general since the foundation of the organization in 1948.

Decision-making in the Assembly is usually by a two-thirds majority, largely controlled by low-income countries through the 'one-state, one-vote' rule and their sheer number. However, high-income countries have the power to influence the WHO agenda through 'voluntary contributions', which account for about 80 per cent of the WHO budget (WHO 2019). As the name implies, voluntary contributions are funds that member countries and other donors provide above and beyond their regular dues to the organization. Unlike the regular budget, these contributions are usually tied to particular programmes or projects.

From its foundation to the present day, the WHO has fulfilled key functions in global health, from the management of international treaties such as the International Health Regulations (IHRs) to the provision of technical assistance to low- and middle-income countries (LMICs) and the coordination of global health programmes. The WHO's most celebrated achievement is arguably the eradication of smallpox in 1980. Today, the WHO is leading global efforts to eradicate polio (confined to Afghanistan and Pakistan) and to reduce malaria incidence and mortality by at least 90 per cent by 2030 (WHO 2015). The WHO also provides normative guidance on various aspects of health and healthcare, developing standards and evaluation tools for health system strengthening, classifying and organizing diseases, and negotiating international agreements to guide and inform state behaviour.

Despite these achievements, the work of the WHO has faced many constraints and challenges, partly arising from its structure and its ambitious global mandate.

First, the WHO budget is too small to fulfil its primary mission of being the 'directing and coordinating authority on international health work' (WHO Constitution, Article 2a). The WHO approved budget for 2020–2021 was only about $4.8 billion (WHO 2019). This has curtailed the autonomy of the organization and its ability to function as implementing agency, both in routine and emergency operations, as the ineffective response to Ebola illustrated (see Chapter 4). After Ebola, the WHO strengthened its response capacity, forming a Health Emergencies Program and launching a Contingency Fund for Emergencies, which can be used to respond rapidly to disease outbreaks and other public health emergencies. Yet these resources are inadequate to address major public health crises, especially when these are protracted over a long period of time such as Covid-19 (WHO 2020b).

Second, as mentioned earlier, the WHO is highly dependent on voluntary contributions, which tend to be skewed towards issues most favoured by donors and may fluctuate as a result of political and economic factors. Notably, in early 2020 the US President Donald J. Trump suspended the payment of voluntary contributions to the WHO, amidst concerns that the organization was 'severely mismanaging and covering up the spread of the coronavirus' (Horton 2020). In July 2020, his administration formally notified the UN that the US would withdraw from the WHO, although this decision was reversed by his successor, President Joe Biden.

Third, a recurrent criticism of the WHO is about the work and effectiveness of the six regional offices, which operate autonomously from the headquarters in Geneva with insufficient oversight and coordination. This problem became evident during the Ebola outbreak, as the African Regional Office (AFRO) did not convene health ministers or open a regional coordination centre until three months after Ebola was confirmed in Guinea (Gostin and Friedman 2015). Furthermore, for political and historical reasons, some member states do not sit within their respective geographical areas, resulting in fragmentation of regional programmes. In Southeast Asia, for example, Thailand and Myanmar are part of the Southeast Asia Regional Office (SEARO), while neighbouring Cambodia, Lao PDR and Vietnam are members of the Western Pacific Regional Office (WPRO).

Lastly, as with other international organizations, the WHO has limited power to enforce compliance with norms and regulations. The IHRs require member states to develop core health capacities to detect and respond to public health emergencies of international concern. The new IHRs entered into force in 2007 and are legally binding, yet compliance remains patchy. It is also worth mentioning that in the early stages of the Covid-19 pandemic the WHO advised member countries to avoid travel restrictions, in line with the approach in the IHRs. However, contrary to the WHO advice, most countries resorted to border closures and flight suspension amidst increasing concerns and domestic political pressure (Ferhani and Rushton 2020).

Other UN agencies

In addition to the WHO, other UN agencies have been involved in global health policy and implementation, including UNICEF, UNDP, the Joint United Nations Program on HIV/AIDS (UNAIDS) and the World Bank. UNICEF was established by the UN General Assembly in December 1946 to support impoverished children in areas devastated by the Second World War. Financed almost entirely by contributions of member states, it has helped feed children in more than 100 countries, providing shelter, healthcare and food. UNICEF's work in health has focused on commodity supply, emergency relief and specialized disease control and eradication programmes. In the early 1960s, UNICEF was involved in the campaign for yaws eradication, which led to a 95% reduction in cases (Asiedu et al. 2008). This success spurred involvement in the campaigns against tuberculosis, trachoma and malaria. Since 2000, much of UNICEF's health work has been guided by the MDGs and, subsequently, the 2030 agenda of the SDGs (Clark et al. 2020).

UNDP is another agency in the UN system that has played an important role in global health, especially in the past two decades. Established in 1965, UNDP has a very similar governance structure to UNICEF with a Secretariat, a 36-member Executive Board and country offices. As the lead UN development agency, UNDP is uniquely placed to help country partners to achieve the SDGs, mobilizing resources and raising awareness. It also serves normative and monitoring functions, publishing the Human Development Report every year, defining measurement tools and standards, and developing policy proposals. UNDP has also worked together with important global health initiatives outside the UN system. In particular, UNDP is a key partner of the Global Fund for HIV/AIDS, TB and Malaria, helping national partners to strengthen capacity for making effective use of the Fund's financing and, in exceptional circumstances, acting as a principal recipient to manage Global Fund grants. UNDP has also been highly influential through its development and promotion of the alternative measure of progress and human well-being: the Human Development Index.

Finally, the UN has responded to the HIV/AIDS epidemic through the establishment of the UNAIDS, a joint programme of cosponsoring agencies (including UNICEF, WHO, UNDP, UNESCO and the World Bank) to advocate and coordinate global action on the HIV/AIDS epidemic. UNAIDS is governed by a Programme Coordinating Board (PCB) that defines and reviews the plan of action and budget for each financial period, with representatives of 22 governments from all geographic regions, the UNAIDS

cosponsoring agencies and representatives of NGOs, including associations of people living with HIV.

UNAIDS has been praised for making NGOs part of its governing body,
managing to get UN agencies to work better together, and its contribution
to epidemiological surveillance data on HIV/AIDS. It has also been praised
for raising the profile of HIV/AIDS and putting it firmly on the global political agenda through advocacy campaigns and resource mobilization. In
2018, however, the reputation of the organization was damaged by an
independent evaluation which described 'a work culture of fear, lack of
trust, and retaliation' (UNAIDS 2018). Following the publication of this
report, the then director Michel Sidibé resigned and calls were made for
reforms to restore confidence in UNAIDS and its ability to maintain leadership of the global effort to end HIV/AIDS as a public health threat.

In sum, the UN system has provided vital support and leadership to
achieve major health and development goals but has also faced many
challenges. Moreover, in the future, the impressive gains made in recent
years – such as the substantial decline in infant and maternal mortality
rates, great progress in HIV response and halving malaria deaths – are
threatened by the effects of the Covid-19 pandemic.

In 2020, the UN annual report on the SDGs warned that Covid-19 will
push millions of people back into extreme poverty and reverse decades of
progress on global health indicators and universal health coverage (UN
2020a). In many LMICs, the direct effects of the pandemic on population
health and the local health systems are compounded by the scaling down
of SDGs funding as donor countries are struggling to recover from the economic effects of Covid-19. Addressing these unprecedented challenges will
require radical innovation in financing for development and the underlying
governance arrangements (UN 2020b).

🖉 Activity 10.2

Think about a global health issue you are particularly interested in. Identify UN agencies that are working on this issue. What is their specific
contribution? Are there differences between their approaches? Do they
collaborate with each other or with the WHO?

Feedback

In addition to the WHO, many specialized agencies in the UN system
have supported a wide range of global health programmes. The involvement of multiple agencies has brought considerable resources and
expertise to address complex health issue such as HIV/AIDS, malaria,
child and maternal health. However, lack of coordination and, at times,

competition between agencies has been a long-standing issue. In recognition of this, specific mechanisms to improve inter-agency cooperation such as UNAIDS have been developed. Another example is the UN Joint Programmes, defined as 'a set of activities contained in a joint work plan and related common budgetary framework, involving two or more UN organizations and (sub) national governmental partners, intended to achieve results aligned with national priorities/mechanisms' (UNDG 2014). In Kenya, for instance, the UN Joint Programme on Reproductive, Maternal, Newborn, Child and Adolescent Health was established to support the government of Kenya and six UN agencies (UNAIDS, UNFPA, UNICEF, WHO, UN Women and the World Bank), working together towards the reduction of preventable maternal, newborn and child deaths.

International economic organizations

The aim of global economic institutions is to create common rules and norms to manage the relations between states, and to create stability, predictability and thus efficiency in the global economy. This includes facilitating trade between states, which can broadly be seen as the remit of the WTO (see also Chapters 2 and 13). The task of creating economic and monetary (i.e. currency exchange rate) stability in the global economy falls principally to the IMF, which offers short-term loans to countries experiencing financial difficulties or temporary dislocations in their domestic economies. The post-2008 global financial crisis has seen the IMF play a role in assisting a number of high-income countries, most notably Greece, as well as LMICs facing the prospect of financial instability. The role of the WB, meanwhile, is to provide funds (principally via loans) and policy advice to support long-term, sustainable economic development, particularly in LMICs. From the outset, the IMF and WB – which are both headquartered in the USA in Washington, DC – were designed to play a complementary role in the management of the global economy. Membership of the WB is also conditional upon membership of the IMF, meaning the membership of the two organizations, which encompass the overwhelming majority of countries in the world, is identical.

Decision-making in the IMF and WB is via a so-called quota system in which voting weights reflect the relative size of national economies and the financial commitments of member states to the organizations, although the organizational norm is to seek consensus on decisions. The United States, the UK, Japan, Germany and France – the five states with the largest voting share within the WB – each appoint their own executive directors. China, the Russian Federation and Saudi Arabia also enjoy permanent representation on the Board of Directors. The remaining 18 positions are elected from the rest of the membership.

By historical convention, rather than any formal legal requirement, the president of the World Bank has been a US national nominated by the US government and the managing director of the IMF has been a European. Thus the leadership and management of these two institutions arguably reflect the interests of the world's wealthiest and most powerful states. This has led to widespread criticism not just of the policies themselves but also in terms of the legitimacy and accountability of the organizations that design and implement them. Had the interests of LMICs been more fully represented, it is argued, some policy failures of the past – such as those associated with the Structural Adjustment Programmes (SAPs) in the 1980s and 1990s, whose effects were felt most clearly in LMICs – could have been avoided (Peet 2009). In particular, the WB and the IMF are often seen as representing a shared ideology that informs the policies they advocate, dubbed the 'Washington Consensus' by commentators. It is argued that this reflects also the predominant position of the US and other high-income countries within the organizations, which promote a broadly neo-liberal agenda focused on fiscal discipline, open markets, deregulation and privatization, which favour these states at the expense of LMICs.

The activities of the IMF and WB have important implications for global health given the structural influence they exert over national economies and their restriction on governments' ability to fund health and other social policies through the 'conditionality' policy that accompanies WM loans – this policy often forced recipient governments to further liberalization and cap public spending on key government sectors, including the health sector. In addition, some of the development activities undertaken by the WB have been explicitly targeted at addressing global health issues – perhaps most notably the HIV/AIDS pandemic in Africa since the 1990s – partly in recognition of poor population health as a key barrier to economic development (Marshall 2008).

Regional integration

Recent decades have seen the emergence of multiple regional governance structures, trade blocs and institutions. The most extensive and developed of these regional entities is the EU, whose internal market is the second largest economy in the world after the United States. Its foundational treaties have created a highly developed, independent legal order and enforcement mechanisms, which extend beyond those of the member states. Its governance structures include not only representatives of member states (who meet at 'the Council') but a permanent civil service ('the Commission') with extensive executive functions and a directly elected Parliament, making it the world's largest and most successful form of transnational representative democracy. Laws in the EU are made through a process of collective decision-making between these institutions whereby proposals ('bills') are drafted by the Commission and amended and adopted by the Council and Parliament jointly. EU laws may also be challenged in national courts and ultimately in the Court of Justice of the European Union (CJEU), whose decisions are binding on member state courts.

In some policy areas, the EU has exclusive law-making and enforcement powers, while in other areas responsibility is shared with member states or is an exclusively 'national' competence. Health policy is an area of shared competence between the EU and member state governments, although the formal health-related powers afforded to the EU in this area are relatively weak, restricted mainly to coordination efforts in public health and reflecting member states' desire to retain control over health services (Greer 2009). However, that does not mean that the EU has been an ineffective or unimportant health actor. While the EU's explicit role in health policy is limited, it has far more extensive powers in the other policy areas that have important health implications, most notably the governance of its single market and trade policy. Decisions taken in these areas have an important structural effect on population health and create a more robust legal basis for regulations to protect citizens' health. For example, it has been through workplace safety and product standards and labelling legislation, under the auspices of the single market, that the EU has had arguably its most significant impact on health.

Perhaps the clearest example of this is tobacco control. Since the 1990s, the Commission has been active in this area through a series of laws (known as directives) related to labelling and product regulation, advertising and sponsorship, and taxation – all of which have been framed as measures to standardize regulation and to improve the functioning of the internal market (McKee et al. 2010). Specific provisions include the 1998 Tobacco Advertising Directive (TAD) (98/43/EC) – and its replacement directive (2003/33/EC) – along with the 2001 and 2014 Tobacco Product Directives (TPDs), which have been subject to legal challenge by the tobacco industry and industry-supportive member states (Holden and Hawkins 2018).

The 2014 TPD contained a range of measures on the content, labelling and packaging of tobacco products and sought to put in place a regulatory framework for electronic cigarettes (e-cigarettes), which had emerged and expanded in use rapidly during the formulation and enactment of the Directive. These measures were then transposed into national law by member states. In some cases, collective action at the EU level forced member states, or created a strong political rationale, for them to go beyond what it would have been politically likely for them to do otherwise. The case of tobacco control demonstrates also the important role of member states' governments and civil society actors in driving forwards the policy agenda with the effect of changing tobacco control laws not just at the national level but across the Union. In this way even relatively small member states, if committed to health, can have widespread effects on health across the EU (see Hawkins et al. 2019). Finally, the size of the EU economy and its ability to enforce common standards across its market means it has a potentially strong regulatory effect on other countries, which may be encouraged or forced to adhere to product standards and many other EU health, environmental and labour standards in order to gain access to the single market. However, the exit of the UK from the EU ('Brexit') has been a prominent reminder that a solid, well-established supranational organization such as the EU remains vulnerable to changing political mood and pressures within member states.

The model of regional integration has been replicated in other areas of the globe in regional organizations such as the African Union (AU). Founded in May 2001, the AU seeks to promote peace, security, stability and economic development on the continent of Africa by creating an institutional framework for the management and settlement of territorial and political disputes between member states and to facilitate the development of common policy initiatives in areas of mutual interest and concern. The issue of health has been central to the AU's mission since its inception with the formation of Aids Watch Africa in 2001, established to coordinate responses to the pandemic across the continent. More recently, in 2017, the AU oversaw the launch of the Africa Centre for Disease Control and Prevention (Africa CDC). Its role also includes the promotion of shared African interests in other global and multilateral forums, institutions and initiatives (e.g. the negotiation of the SDGs) or within the WTO. In addition, the AU has permanent observer status at the UN General Assembly and maintains a diplomatic mission to the US and the EU. Unlike the EU, the AU is not based on a single internal market as its keystone project but instead seeks to play a coordinating function between the eight regional economic blocs which have emerged in the continent.

In other parts of the world, more overtly economic regional blocs have emerged, including the Association of South-East Asian Nations (ASEAN), the Asia-Pacific Economic Co-operation (APEC), the Common Market of the South (Mercado Común del Sur; MERCOSUR) in Southern America and the United States Mexico Canada Agreement (USMCA, formerly NAFTA). These much looser associations of states focus on trade facilitation and the liberalization of trade barriers (i.e. the removal of tariff and non-tariff trade barriers; see Chapter 13). As part of these processes, they may also coordinate public health cooperation between member countries and, at times, members may act collectively or represent shared interests in other multilateral forums. However, the specific details of these agreements – and the degree of integration and interdependence that they imply – vary greatly, so each agreement should be examined in its own terms and evaluated independently.

✎ Activity 10.3

Choose an international or regional organization of interest to you. Write one or two paragraphs explaining why member states would seek to join, and how they are affected by their membership of your chosen organization. Address the following questions in your answer:

1. In what ways are states able to use these institutions to achieve their health policy aims and objectives?
2. How can they influence decision-making? Are some states more able to do this than others?
3. How might membership of these organizations limit their ability to achieve their health policy aims?

Feedback

States may be affected in a number of ways by their membership of IGOs. International organizations place obligations on states but also confer certain rights. The ability of states to influence these organizations and to pursue their aims and objectives through them will depend on both the formal governance mechanisms of the organization and the *de facto modus operandi*. For example, in the IMF/WB voting rights explicitly recognize the asymmetry of states in terms of economic size and power in their decision-making systems. Similarly, the UN Security Council gives a veto to its five permanent members. Other UN agencies (and the WTO) operate on a consensus-based decision-making model. While, formally, these work on the basis of 'one member, one vote', in reality, the decisions they reach are often the result of power politics. As such, larger, richer states may dictate the terms of the deals struck and the rules enforced.

In addition, the ability of states to enact certain domestic policies may be curtailed by the obligations they have entered into in a certain IGO. This includes commitments under global trade agreements and environmental measures such as the Paris Climate Accord, which requires governments to cut emissions and this may have knock-on effects on their ability to pursue certain domestic policies. For example, the Australian government's decision to introduce plain packaging for tobacco products was challenged under the WTO law and could have resulted in the measures being struck down (see Chapter 13).

Summary

This chapter provided an overview of different types of agreements and institutional arrangements that have been established to enable cooperation between states, including in the area of health. While states remain the main actors in the international arena – particularly the largest, most powerful states – these developments have shaped global health as a field of policy and practice as new modes of governance at the regional and global level were introduced. Since the mid-2010s, however, the resurgence of political and economic nationalism in Europe, the United States and Brazil has led to a crisis of multilateralism and regional cooperation, which poses a direct threat to these institutions and their legitimacy, with potentially far-reaching negative implications for the pursuit of the common good in health and in other policy areas (Morrison 2018). Brexit in the UK and the withdrawal of the US from WHO under President Trump are two symptoms of this political process. The economic impact of the coronavirus on the UN system and financing for global health and development is another important phenomenon, which may reverse progress towards the achievement of the SDGs and universal health coverage. It is perhaps still too early to assess the public health impact of these disruptions, but these are certainly issues that deserve close and constant scrutiny from all stakeholders involved.

References

Asiedu, K., Amouzou, B., Dhariwal, A. et al. (2008) Yaws eradication: past efforts and future perspectives, *Bulletin of the World Health Organization*, 86(7): 499.

Chan, M. (2012) Universal coverage is the ultimate expression of fairness. Acceptance speech at the 65th World Health Assembly, Geneva, Switzerland, 23 May.

Clark, H., Coll-Seck, A.M., Banerjee, A. et al. (2020) A future for the world's children? A WHO-UNICEF-Lancet Commission, *The Lancet*, 395(10224): 605–658. Available at: https://doi.org/10.1016/S0140-6736(19)32540-1.

Cueto, M., Brown, T. and Fee, E. (2019) *The World Health Organization: A History*. Cambridge: Cambridge University Press.

Evertz, S. (2010) *How Ideology Trumped Science: Why PEPFAR Has Failed to Meet Its Potential*. Washington, DC: Center for American Progress.

Ferhani, A. and Rushton, S. (2020) The International Health Regulations, Covid-19, and bordering practices: who gets in, what gets out, and who gets rescued?, *Contemporary Security Policy*, 41(3): 458–477. Available at: https://doi.org/10.1080/13523260.2020.1771955.

Gostin, L.O. and Friedman, E.A. (2015) A retrospective and prospective analysis of the west African Ebola virus disease epidemic: robust national health systems at the foundation and an empowered WHO at the apex, *The Lancet*, 385(9980): 1902–1909. Available at: https://doi.org/10.1016/S0140-6736(15)60644-4.

Greer, S. (2009) *The Politics of European Union Health Policies*. Maidenhead: Open University Press.

Hanhimäki, J.M. (2105) *The United Nations: A Very Short Introduction*, 2nd edn. Oxford: Oxford University Press.

Hawkins, B., Holden, C. and Mackinder, S. (2019) *The Battle for Standardised Cigarette Packaging in Europe: Multi-level Governance, Policy Transfer and the Integrated Strategy of the Global Tobacco Industry*. Basingstoke: Palgrave Macmillan.

Holden, C. and Hawkins, B. (2018) Law, market building and public health in the European Union, *Global Social Policy*, 18(1): 45–61. Available at: https://doi.org/10.1177/1468018117745689.

Horton, R. (2020) Why President Trump is wrong about WHO, *Lancet*, 395(10233): 1330. Available at: https://doi.org/10.1016/S0140-6736(20)30969-7.

Jarman, H. (2015) *The Politics of Trade and Tobacco Control*. Basingstoke: Palgrave Macmillan.

Marshall, K. (2008) *The World Bank: From Reconstruction to Development to Equity*. London: Routledge.

Marten, R. (2018) How states exerted power to create the Millennium Development Goals and how this shaped the global health agenda, *Global Public Health*, 14(4): 584–599.

McKee, M., Hervey, T. and Gilmore, A. (2010) Public health policies, in Mossialos, E., Baeten, R., Permanand, G. et al. (eds) *Health Systems Governance in Europe: The Role of European Union Law and Policy*. Cambridge: Cambridge University Press.

Morrison, J.S. (2018) Global health disruptors: Decay of the post-war multilateral Western order, *The BMJ Opinion*. Available at: https://blogs.bmj.com/bmj/2018/11/29/stephen-morrison-decay-of-the-postwar-multilateral-western-order/ (accessed 9 April 2021).

Peet, R. (2009) *Unholy Trinity: The IMF, World Bank and WTO*, 2nd edn. London: Zed Books.

UN (2020a) *The Sustainable Development Goals Report*. Available at: https://unstats.un.org/sdgs/report/2020/The-Sustainable-Development-Goals-Report-2020.pdf (accessed 21 April 2021).

UN (2020b) *Financing for Development in the Era of Covid-19 and Beyond: Menu of Options for the Consideration of Heads of State and Government* (Part I). Available at: https://globalization.un.org/sites/un2.un.org/files/financing_for_development_covid19_part_i_hosg.pdf (accessed 21 April 2021).

UNAIDS (2018) Report on the work of the Independent Expert Panel on Prevention of and response to harassment, including sexual harassment; bullying and abuse of power at UNAIDS Secretariat. Geneva: Joint United Nations Programme on HIV/AIDS. Available at: http://globalization.unaids.org/sites/default/files/media_asset/report-iep_en.pdf (cited 6 January 2019).

UNDG (2014) *Guidance Note on Joint Programmes*. New York: United Nations Development Group. Available at: https://unsdg.un.org/resources/undg-guidance-note-joint-programmes (accessed 9 April 2021).

US Department of State (USDS) (2021) *US President's Emergency Plan for AIDS Relief (PEPFAR)*. Available at: https://globalization.state.gov/pepfar/. Available at: https://globalization.state.gov/pepfar/ (accessed 9 April 2021).

WHO (1948) *Constitution of the World Health Organization*. Geneva: WHO. Available at: apps.who.int/gb/bd/PDF/bd47/EN/constitution-en.pdf (accessed 9 April 2021).

WHO (1978) Declaration of Alma-Ata. International Conference on Primary Health Care, Alma-Ata, USSR, 6–12 September 1978. Geneva: World Health Organization. Available at: https://www.who.int/publications/almaata_declaration_en.pdf (accessed 8 November 2021).

WHO (2015) *Global Technical Strategy for Malaria 2016–2030*. Geneva: World Health Organization.

WHO (2019) *Programme Budget 2020–2021*. Geneva: World Health Organization. Available at: https://globalization.who.int/about/finances-accountability/budget/WHOPB-PRP-19.pdf?ua=1 (accessed 9 April 2021).

WHO (2020) *Independent Oversight and Advisory Committee for the WHO Health Emergencies Programme*. Geneva: World Health Organization.

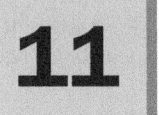

11 Commercial actors in global health

Benjamin Hawkins

Overview

This chapter examines the impact of the commercial sector on global health and the involvement of commercial actors in global health governance. Commercial actors, such as transnational corporations, are economically powerful and politically influential and their activities have significant effects on population health. Thus, any account of the field of global health governance (GHG) that ignores the commercial sector is incomplete. This chapter addresses the role played by commercial actors in the production of ill health, their role in healthcare provision and the various ways in which they attempt to influence health governance arrangements at the national and global levels. It focuses principally on the examples of the global tobacco and alcohol industries, but the market and political strategies identified in these sectors are more widely evident.

Learning objectives

After working through this chapter, you will be able to:

- Define the commercial sector and differentiate it from other global health actors.
- Describe ways in which commercial actors impact on population health.
- Assess the nature of commercial power in the context of globalization.
- Evaluate the roles played by commercial actors in global health governance.
- Critically assess the motivation behind companies' corporate social responsibility programmes.

Key terms

The commercial sector: The body of private sector, profit-making entities such as businesses and corporations, and the organizations that support their activities such as trade associations and lobbyists.

Transnational corporations (TNCs): A corporation is an association of stockholders that is regarded as a 'legal person' under most national laws.

Transnational corporations are those economically active across national boundaries, often in many countries across the globe.

Regulation: The enforcement of norms, standards, rules and principles that govern behaviour.

Corporate social responsibility: Industry-supported measures whereby companies attempt to demonstrate responsible behaviour in their core business practices or to be good corporate citizens through activities such as philanthropic donations.

Defining the commercial sector

When we talk about the *commercial sector*, we are referring to private actors, such as *corporations* that exist explicitly to produce profits. The commercial sector also includes a range of associated organizations that are established to support a particular *firm* or *industry*. These may include *business federations* or *trade associations*, such as the International Federation of Pharmaceutical Manufacturers Associations (IFPMA) or the International Chambers of Commerce (ICC). Other groups, which appear to be unrelated to the commercial sector, may actually be funded and controlled by industry actors to promote a particular policy agenda favourable to their interests. For example, The Institute of Regulatory Policy was funded by Philip Morris to lobby the US government on tobacco control issues (Muggli et al. 2004). The defining feature of the commercial sector is its market orientation and the pursuit of profit. As such, they can be differentiated from non-governmental organizations (NGOs) and other civil society bodies such as professional associations (e.g. the Royal Colleges in the UK) or trade unions (see Chapter 12). Thus, while commercial actors may have additional societal, environmental or other objectives – which may feature prominently in corporate messaging, advertising and in their online and social media presences – these are necessarily secondary to the underlying search for profit. Indeed, they are often designed to support commercial objectives by generating a positive brand image for companies or to counter criticism about their societal or environmental impact (Mialon and McCambridge 2018; Dorfman et al. 2012).

The increasing movement of goods, services, people and capital between states that has occurred as a result of globalization has been characterized also by significant growth in the number and scale of global firms which seek to take advantage of new opportunities for profit brought about by these processes (Gleeson and Labonte 2020). In the context of global health policy, we often focus on transnational corporations (TNCs) such as those in the tobacco, alcohol and food sectors, active in multiple countries, as 'commercial determinants' of health with significant ability to affect health outcomes and to influence regulatory regimes and policy debates (McKee and Stuckler 2018). It is these TNCs, within the wider commercial sector, which will be the focus of this chapter. The term multinational corporation is also used in the literature and, for the purposes of this chapter, can be seen as identical to a TNC.

A key feature of corporations is that they have the status of a 'legal person' (sometimes referred to as an 'artificial person') independent of their ownership, which means corporations enjoy specific rights and legal protections. This includes the ability to use courts and other arbitration forums, both domestically and internationally, to sue in order to guarantee their rights. Corporations' attempts to protect their rights – for example, the intellectual property rights of pharmaceutical companies and tobacco companies – are at the centre of many current debates in global health governance (see Chapter 13). Meanwhile, stockholders have what lawyers' term 'limited liability' for the activities and debts incurred by the company.

✏ Activity 11.1

Make a list of *three* reasons why health policymakers should pay attention to the role(s) of the commercial sector in global health governance. In framing your response, consider the nature of global health problems, the capacity of the state to address them and the assets of the commercial sector.

Feedback

Your answer might include (but may not be limited to) the following considerations:

- Commercial actors are intimately involved in the creation of ill health (e.g. through selling unhealthy goods like tobacco and through environmental degradation).
- They are also central to the provision of health services and treatment, through the development and manufacture of medical devices, drugs and the health system architecture (e.g. hospitals).
- The health impacts of transborder flows often exceed the regulatory capacity of governments, whether acting alone or collectively through inter-governmental organizations. These challenges include:
  - The (legitimate and illicit) trade in goods and services and the movement of persons across borders
  - The spread of antimicrobial resistance, pathogens and infectious diseases, environmental pollution and population migration

- Since the commercial sector (along with other actors) often plays a key role in the flow of people and things across borders, there have been calls to rethink classical, state-centric public health approaches to dealing with them. This has included an increasing tendency for policymakers to work in partnership with the commercial sector and to draw on their expertise, resources and logistical capacity. Commercial actors are often involved in the governance of health issues, particularly those arising from their activities in ways that they argue can contribute to public health goals.
- The involvement of corporations in policymaking raises questions about the effectiveness of industry self-regulation and about the potential conflicts of interest that arise from industry involvement in policymaking and delivery.
- Corporations' economic power and their role as political actors in global health governance make them impossible to ignore.

Corporations and the provision of healthcare

One way in which the commercial sector is of relevance to global health is through activities that promote health or deliver healthcare. Corporations may be the direct providers of many core health services, such as residential care homes for the elderly, optometry practices and private hospitals. As well as services, they produce a range of goods and technologies required to diagnose and treat illnesses, such as scanning machines and medications. At times, this necessitates the close cooperation between the public and private sector to develop new treatments and technologies. This was evident for example in the collective efforts of governments, universities and the pharmaceutical industry in their response to the Covid-19 pandemic and the move to develop and bring to market a number of vaccines in unprecedented speed. In many countries, corporations are providers of health insurance and are involved in the financing and construction of the health service infrastructure. In certain contexts, corporations may become involved in the distribution of medicines through established supply chains which extend into areas where the infrastructure of the state may be unable to fully or effectively govern a particular territory. This may be the case in remote locations in low- and middle-income countries (LMICs) or in conflict and post-conflict settings.

For example, in 2018 the Global Fund announced a partnership with the brewer Heineken, which was justified in part on the ability of Heineken's cold storage transportation network to deliver medications requiring refrigeration to destinations in Africa. Despite the apparent rationale for this, the Global Fund was widely criticized for the conflict of interest involved in working with the alcohol industry, given the role of alcohol as a structural driver of HIV infection (Marten and Hawkins 2018) and the questionable business practices of the company in the continent (van Beeman 2019).

Finally, corporations play a significant role in the health and well-being of those they employ by providing safe working environments and support for employees suffering from physical and mental illnesses. In the context of globalization, health services as well as healthcare equipment are being traded across borders requiring transnational regulatory and governance regimes. As such, the trade in both goods and health services becomes a global health issue (Baum and Anaf 2015).

Corporations and the production of ill health

The activities of transnational corporations producing tobacco, alcoholic beverages and foods high in sugar, salt and fat are associated with a number of chronic diseases, which are now the principal causes of death in high-income countries and, increasingly, they are also impacting LMICs (see Chapters 3 and 6). Corporations in these sectors employ sophisticated marketing and promotional strategies to sell their products, driving consumption and with this health harms. At the same time their corporate political strategies are designed to create favourable regulatory environments for their businesses, for example through avoidance of taxation or restrictions on their ability to sell or advertise their brands (Moodie et al. 2013).

Tobacco industry actors are singled out for special treatment and largely excluded from policymaking at the country and global levels including specific provisions in Article 5.3 of the WHO Framework Convention on Tobacco Control (FCTC) requiring signatory governments to take explicit steps to prevent their undue influence over policy (Fooks et al. 2017; see also Chapter 9). The pariah status of the tobacco industry is in part a result of the level of knowledge we have about their activities through the release of internal industry documents following litigation in the USA in the 1990s (Hurt et al. 2009). Much of the academic literature and the policy discourse surrounding tobacco control treats the product and the industry that produces it as a special case, given the uniquely harmful nature of tobacco and the often covert tactics employed by the tobacco industry to defend their interests (Casswell 2013). For example, the United Nations (UN) High Meeting on the Prevention and Control of Non-Communicable Diseases precluded engagement with the tobacco industry while welcoming partnerships with other industry actors, including the food and alcohol industries (Moodie et al. 2013).

While not underplaying the harmful nature of smoking and the mendacity of the tobacco industry, recent studies of the alcohol and other sectors such as the processed food and beverage industries have sought to problematize this idea of tobacco 'exceptionalism' (Hawkins et al. 2018a). Identifying both the significant levels of harm associated with these products and the similarities in the structure and strategies of the industries that sell and promote them, public health actors have begun to argue that we should extend the same regulatory approach and give the same level of scrutiny to corporate actors in other industries.

As firms expand their reach, there is an increasing need for rules to govern their transactions on a global basis. International regimes and global regulations do have certain advantages for transnational corporations. They minimize uncertainty, create common standards allowing the production of uniform products that can be sold in markets across the globe and reduce transaction costs. However, global regulations may also present challenges to these global companies, as is the case with the FCTC. Global action in this instance established a consensus on 'best practice' in tobacco control and sought to marginalize tobacco companies in health policymaking (Matthes et al. 2020). This created a powerful normative basis for tobacco control advocates in countries across the globe to advocate for stricter tobacco control policies and to hold government to account for the commitments they had made. As this demonstrates, in the context of globalization, decisions taken at one level may affect those at another.

Analysing corporate power

It is useful to think of corporate power in the context of global health governance in terms of structure and agency (Farnsworth and Holden 2006). Structural power is derived from the privileged position capital owners occupy in the market economy. Agency power is based on direct social relations and refers to the deliberate exercise of influence.

Structural power

Structural power is based on control over investment. A state may be dependent on the revenue generated by the activities of a corporation, the foreign direct investment it provides and/or the employment it creates. An obvious example of this is the duty paid on cigarettes or alcohol, which have proved major barriers towards effective regulation of these industries as finance ministries fear the loss of revenue from lower levels of consumption of these products. Similarly, governments may be sympathetic to the case of pharmaceutical companies who provide employment, corporation tax revenues and, not least, life-saving medicines.

It can be argued that the structural power of corporations has increased in the context of globalization, because it has provided transnational corporations with the 'capacity for exit'. In other words, they are able to relocate from one country to another to seek more favourable conditions (e.g. the tax regime or subsidies and other incentives offered by governments) (Farnsworth and Holden 2006). The effect of relocation is a loss of corporation tax revenue and potentially even more wide-reaching effects in terms of economic growth, employment, public spending and welfare costs. In countries where the government is reliant on a single industry or even a single corporation for the majority of its income, the threat of exit is a powerful tool.

Corporations also have ideological influence over governments and citizens. Within much of the world, and particularly in high-income countries, there is a high level of acceptance for the pro-business ideas popularized by corporate actors favouring free markets, deregulation and low levels of taxation. In many contexts, particularly in advanced industrial economies in the Global North such as the US, the UK and Europe where many of the largest TNCs are headquartered, business leaders and the private sector are often venerated as the engine of economic growth and creators of employment and tax revenues. The result of this is that it is seen as acceptable for corporations to be present in ever-expanding areas of public life, including in the development and implementation of public policy.

Agency power

Agency power may take the form of political engagement, such as lobbying governments, regulatory bodies and international organizations, or through related activities such as the funding of political parties or campaigns for office. However, there are subtler and less obvious processes through which corporations act to further their interests. One way of doing this is participation in various institutions and agencies involved in the formulation or delivery of policy and through self-regulatory or co-regulatory regimes. In addition, corporations may be involved in government committees or state delegations to international organizations or trade negotiations. For example, representatives of transnational pharmaceutical company, Pfizer, served in the US delegation which negotiated the formation of the World Trade Organization (WTO) and the inclusion within this of the controversial Agreement on Trade Related Aspects of Intellectual Property (TRIPS), which enabled companies to more effectively protect their commercial patents, but may have reduced access to essential medicines (Sell 2003; see Chapter 13).

In this way, the attempts by corporations to influence the policy process may focus on all levels of that process: local, national, regional (for example, the EU) and even global. Their presence in these forums is in large part the result of their attempts to depict themselves as 'stakeholders' in the policy process, with particular expertise in a certain sector, which enables them to contribute to the formulation of good policies and the ability to oversee their effective implementation on the ground. TNCs that understand the dynamic of multi-level governance may seek to shift decision-making to the level or the arena in which they are most effectively or efficiently able to achieve their desired outcome: a process known as venue shifting (see Hawkins and Holden 2016; Holden and Hawkins 2018).

Economic power

In addition to the involvement of corporations in both the production and treatment of ill health, their economic strength means they are simply too large and important a group of actors to ignore. Indeed, the economic resources of the world's largest TNCs often dwarf those of international organizations and even states. For example, the decision of cigarette company Philip Morris International to use international trade and investment law to sue the government of Uruguay, a country of around 3 million people, over its introduction of increased cigarette packet warning labels placed significant economic pressure on the country to defend its case and its legal costs were eventually covered by the American billionaire and health campaigner, Michael Bloomberg (Lencucha 2010; Hawkins and Holden 2016). This provides a stark example of the relative economic power of corporations and even individuals compared to many countries. The economic strength of transnational corporations means they also wield formidable political strength, since this economic power affords them high degrees of access to, and potentially influence over, policymakers at the local, national and supranational levels.

Influencing global health governance

Corporations can exert influence over policymaking at the national as well as the global level and at all points during the policymaking and governance process (see, for example, Hawkins and McCambridge 2020). They will look to use all available channels through which they can engage either the officials involved in the drafting of legislation or parliamentarians who will enact it into law. Equally, once laws are in place, there is often substantial debate about the way in which they are to be implemented and enforced and how their impacts are to be evaluated, which industry actors can seek to influence. A range of corporate influencing tactics are set out in Box 11.1.

Box 11.1   Corporate influencing strategies

- Agenda setting and issue management. Seeking to shape public discourses and policy debates to keep unfavoured issues off the policy agenda. For example, framing sugar taxes as an affront to personal freedom and choice to make them politically controversial (Dorfman et al. 2012).

- Blocking the adoption of new laws or measures. The use of political lobbying and other influencing strategies to stop new laws being adopted (see McCambridge et al. 2018).
- Influencing the content of a policy instrument. If it is impossible to stop the adoption of unfavoured measures, then seek to influence the specific form and content. For example, tobacco companies lobbied at the national and international levels to secure changes to the text of the Framework Convention on Tobacco Control (Grüning et al. 2012; see also Chapter 9).
- Challenge or delay the implementation of a policy measure. For example, the tobacco industry sought to prevent the adoption of standardized packaging measures for tobacco in Australia and Europe through a range of legal challenges (Hawkins and Holden 2016; Hawkins et al. 2018b; Jarman 2013; see also Chapter 13).
- Challenging the credibility/validity of the instruments. For example, the global alcohol industry represented by bodies such as the Scotch Whisky Association has repeatedly challenged the internationally accepted evidence base on the effectiveness of minimum pricing to reduce alcohol-related harm (McCambridge et al. 2013).
- Undermining the legitimacy and capacity of an international organization charged with negotiating an instrument. For example, it is reported that Philip Morris undertook the largest lobbying campaign ever mounted in order to 'block, amend and delay' the 2014 European Union (EU) Tobacco Products Directive (TPD) (Hawkins et al. 2018b; Peeters et al. 2016).
- Challenging the competence of a UN body to develop norms in a particular domain. For example, the food industry has tried to circumscribe the extent to which WHO can address obesity by proposing policies and regulations (Waxman 2004).

Delivering 'policy goods'

The expertise possessed by corporations is a crucial resource of power as this is often invaluable to policymakers supporting corporations' claims to be key stakeholders in the policy process. In some areas, such as the technological sector or with new product innovations, corporations are often the main (or even only) source of key technical expertise in a given area. In the alcohol sector, for example, corporations have particular specialism in packaging design and also in advertising and marketing, which may be valuable to governments in designing health warning labels or public information campaign (Mialon and McCambridge 2018). However, the involvement of such actors in the design of policy measures comes with the risk of a conflict of interest (COI) since the objectives of the industry – to sell more of a product such as alcohol – run counter to the aims of warning labels of health messaging which seek to encourage consumers to reduce their consumption to protect their health (Ralston et al. 2021; Gilmore and Fooks 2012). Consequently, industry actors may engage with government in ways that formally appear supportive of their policy goals but may do so in ways that actually seek to minimize their effectiveness.

Self-regulation

In addition to influencing global health governance, many corporations advocate the advantages of self-regulation over government legislation or compulsorily regulations. There are two principal types of self-regulation: regulating 'market standards' and 'social standards'. In practice, however, it can be difficult to distinguish between self-regulation of market and social standards, as some mechanisms pursue both goals (Moodie et al. 2013). In the case of market standards, products, process and business practice may be subject to governance to support commerce (e.g. to reduce transaction costs or increase confidence in a product). Although such self-regulation may have social impacts, the overriding purpose of market standards is to enable commerce.

By contrast, self-regulation through social standards involves business and industry voluntarily adopting and observing specific practices based on public or social concern rather than to improve the functioning of the market. Self-regulatory social standards are usually developed in response to consumer concerns or boycotts, shareholder activism or the threat of impending public regulation. Self-regulation of social standards occurs through mechanisms including voluntary codes and reporting initiatives, statements of principles, guidelines and codes of practice, and some public–private partnerships as well as corporate social responsibility activities (discussed below). Self-regulatory initiatives often address issues that are already subject to (often ineffective) statutory regulation. For example, the International Labour Organization (ILO) has issued standards governing maternity leave and breastfeeding at work. However, not all countries have adopted the standards, while implementation is often partial even in those states that have formally adopted the measures.

It can be argued that self-regulation and voluntary codes of practice can bring new stakeholders into the regulatory process. For example, temporary and informal labourers, often women, have participated in developing workplace codes, having not typically been represented in comparable ILO processes (Agarwala 2007; Jones 2012). Second, codes may generate better compliance than public regulation. Experience with many international conventions governing social and economic issues suggests that ratifying governments often fail to implement them but cannot be held accountable by the international community for such failure. In theory, companies adopt codes to gain market share and comply with them to retain the confidence of their consumers/shareholders. Third, codes are less costly to the public sector than statutory regulation.

There are many reasons for scepticism regarding the ability of voluntary codes to adequately govern many global health issues. The codes often comprise lofty statements of intent but lack the means to ensure delivery on their commitment or sufficient transparency to allow effective monitoring. Consequently, such patchwork self-regulation may result in 'enclave' social policy, governing select issues and groups of workers at specific points in their working lives. Since codes of practice are voluntary, they are not traceable to public authority and cannot be legally enforced. Thus, they may erode societal commitment to universal, legally enforceable rights and entitlements.

✐ Activity 11.2

Why might a company commit itself to adhering to a voluntary code? Suggest four to five reasons why this may be advantageous to them.

Feedback

While serving social purposes, codes can serve important business functions and ultimately increase profits. Your answer should also include some of the following reasons why voluntary codes may be adopted by a company:

- To demonstrate responsiveness to societal concerns.
- To provide material for public relations.
- To differentiate itself from competitors to increase sales.
- To respond to concerns of consumers to increase sales.
- To respond to concerns of shareholders and encourage greater investment.
- To decrease costs. The British mining conglomerate, Anglo American PLC, estimates that 30,000 of its employees in South Africa are infected with HIV. It has voluntarily adopted a code in relation to treatment of 3000 employees, costs being reportedly offset by sharp declines in mortality and absenteeism due to illness.
- To stave off or delay statutory regulation. The tobacco, pharmaceutical and food safety codes mentioned above were advanced to pre-empt more onerous international obligations.
- To provide flexible tools tailored to specific problems instead of blanket regulations covering all contingencies.

Co-regulation

In other areas of policy, the aims and objectives of commercial actors may not be to influence the content of particular laws or policies, but to position themselves as partners in the delivery of certain policy measures. This amounts to a deal between public authorities and private sector organizations, often involving civil society as well as corporate actors. While examples of co-regulator regimes are common at the national level, the most obvious example of this type of governance structure at the global level is the UN Global Compact (see Box 11.2).

Box 11.2   Case study: The UN Global Compact

The UN Global Compact is the first attempt to regulate the activities of transnational corporations at the global level via the UN. It set out a number of principles to guide the conduct of corporations and ensure they act in compliance with a set of ethical standards relating to human rights, labour standards, environmental protection and the fight against corruption. These include commitments to do the following:

- Support and respect the protection of internationally proclaimed human rights.
- Ensure they are not complicit in human rights abuses.
- Uphold the freedom of association and the effective recognition of the right to collective bargaining.
- Eliminate all forms of forced and compulsory labour.
- Abolish child labour.
- Eliminate discrimination in employment.
- Support a precautionary approach to environmental challenges.
- Undertake initiatives to promote greater environmental responsibility.
- Encourage the development and diffusion of environmentally friendly technologies.
- Ensure businesses work against all forms of corruption, including extortion and bribery.

Supporters of the Compact argue that, in the context of globalization, in which national governments and inter-governmental organizations struggle to effectively regulate the cross-border activities of TNCs, it offers an innovative form of governance that attempts to create new accountability mechanisms. While these may be weaker than more robust forms of regulation and enforcement at the national level, this reflects the 'anarchic' nature of the global sphere and the absence of an effective world government able to police transnational corporate activity.

> The Compact has been criticized for being voluntary and largely unenforceable, while offering the mark of respectability to companies. These include corporations active in controversial industries, such as the oil and tobacco industries, although in the case of British American Tobacco, their overtures have to date been rebuffed.
>
> In addition, the Compact has been criticized as undermining more robust forms of regulation. While the hope of the UN was to 'fill a void between regulatory regimes, at one end of the spectrum, and voluntary codes of industry, at the other' (Global Compact Office, 2002: 4), in practice, the Compact reinforces 'the pendulum swing away from stricter forms of regulation' (Utting 2002).

Co-regulation presents a third way between traditional public, statutory regulation and private self-regulation. It can be seen as a degree of involvement of the public sector (government) in processes of business self-regulation. It has arisen due to the inadequacies of public and private regulation. The former, it has been argued, is inadequate in an era of globalization as state and inter-governmental capacity for regulation lags behind technological advances made by industry. Furthermore, it can be difficult for national governments to enforce national regimes unilaterally, and global regulatory regimes are difficult to achieve and even harder to enforce.

The idea is that the public and private sector negotiate on an agreed set of policy or regulatory objectives that are results oriented. Subsequently, the private sector takes responsibility for implementation of the provisions. Monitoring compliance may remain a public responsibility or otherwise be contracted out to a third party – sometimes an interested non-governmental organization. The advent of co-regulation is relatively new, and there has been more formal experimentation with it at the national and regional levels. The European Union, for example, is experimenting with co-regulation particularly with respect to the internet, journalism and e-commerce. The UN's Global Compact with industry might be viewed as a form of co-regulation, together with many of the global public–private partnerships (PPPs).

Corporate social responsibility

Corporate social responsibility (CSR) is a loose umbrella term incorporating a diverse set of measures undertaken by companies to improve the impact their activities have on the social environments in which they are present. A more cynical interpretation of CSR may conclude that its main objective is not to change corporate behaviour or the impact of this but to change the perception of that behaviour among governments and the general public. In the case of the former, CSR may be seen as an attempt to ward off further regulation of the industry or to buttress existing self-regulatory regimes that are favourable to the business. In the case of the latter, CSR may work to improve the image of a corporation in the minds of consumers, to set it aside from competitors, and to win customers on the basis of its ethical or responsible business policies. There has been a rapid expansion of interest in CSR in recent years in response to a huge increase in corporate focus in this area. This in turn may be seen as a response to increased concern about environmental sustainability and the social impact of corporate activity among consumers and mounting criticism of some corporate behaviour. In broad terms, CSR may be considered as a strategy that might serve three types of company:

- Those with social and environmental principles genuinely at the core of their business; examples of this type of company include the Cooperative Bank, which places a great emphasis on its ethical lending and investment policies.
- Corporations aiming to create a link between their brand and social responsibility programmes via partnerships and joint marketing activities. An example here is the football team FC Barcelona, which carried the UNICEF logo on its jersey.
- Controversial industries that are responding to pressure from consumers, investors or regulators. This includes the tobacco and alcohol industries, as well as other controversial industries such as those implicated in environmental degradation and climate change, for example the fossil fuel and automotive industries.

There is evidence that tobacco corporations saw CSR measures focusing on environmental protection and the eradication of child labour in the field of tobacco cultivation as being important ways through which they are able to repair their image and fend off calls for still further regulation of their markets (Fooks et al. 2011). Meanwhile transnational alcohol companies, particularly in water-intensive sectors such as beer brewing, have associated themselves with initiatives to provide clean drinking water in Africa at precisely the moment they began to enter or expand their presence in African markets, with implications for local water supplies (Hanefeld et al. 2016).

✎ **Activity 11.3**

Imagine you are the CEO of a multinational alcoholic drinks retailer. Faced with rising levels of alcohol consumption and falling prices, the government is seeking to introduce a minimum price for alcohol to be sold, which you oppose. How might you go about opposing this?

Feedback

Your answer might include the following strategies. You may attempt to frame the policy debate and shape perceptions of the problem of alcohol related harm, as well as the effectiveness of minimum pricing as an intervention to address this through media campaigns. You may promote studies and other evidence that supports this position (or promotes your favoured alternative interventions). You may even fund studies by sympathetic researchers or think tanks, which undermine the rationale for pricing policy or show it to be ineffective. You may attempt to keep the issue of pricing, or alcohol policy more generally, off the policy agenda through relationship building or lobby influential politicians or those with industry connections (e.g. with industry installations such bottling plants in their areas). You could seek to deflect attention from alcohol pricing by suggesting less effective alternatives that would not have such a large impact on sales, such as public education campaign or self- and co-regulatory regimes. If you cannot keep alcohol pricing off the agenda you will lobby government ministers, aides and parliamentarians to try to stop any new laws passing. If the attempt to block these laws is unsuccessful and they do pass, you may seek to prevent or delay their implementation through legal challenges and seek to reverse or repeal the policy even after it has been enacted. This may include seeking to undermine the policy by influencing its evaluation and undermining perceptions of its effectiveness. In reviewing your answer, consult the publications by McCambridge et al. (2014) and Hawkins and McCambridge (2021), which examine this case and Hawkins et al. (2018a), which discusses alcohol industry strategy more generally. See also Chapter 13 on trade agreements and how they are used by corporations to challenge unfavoured public health measures.

Summary

In summary, this chapter has explored the role of corporations as incredibly powerful economic and political actors that play an active role in almost every aspect of global health policy. There is a wide range of mechanisms open to corporations and an equally wide range of tactics they employ to influence policy. In recent decades, their influence has increased in line with underlying ideological shifts in society and an increasingly firm commitment to neo-liberal ideas about the effectiveness of markets and private sector actors in delivering social goods. However, the move towards co-regulation and self-regulation, which this ideological shift has ushered in, raises a number of issues about accountability and effectiveness. It raises questions about whether corporate actors should be involved in setting the rules that govern them, and the consequences of this for global health.

References

Agarwala, R. (2007) Resistance and compliance in the age of globalization: Indian women and labor organizations, *The Annals of the American Academy of Political and Social Science*, 610: 143–159. Available at: http://globalization.jstor.org/stable/25097891 (accessed 25 June 2021).

Baum, F.E. and Anaf, J.M. (2015) Transnational corporations and health: a research agenda, *International Journal of Health Services*, 45(2): 353–362.

Casswell, S. (2013) Vested interests in addiction research and policy. Why do we not see the corporate interests of the alcohol industry as clearly as we see those of the tobacco industry?, *Addiction*, 108(4): 680–685.

Dorfman, L., Cheyne, A., Friedman, L.C. et al. (2012) Soda and tobacco industry corporate social responsibility campaigns: how do they compare?, *PLoS Medicine*, 9(6): e1001241.

Farnsworth, K. and Holden, C. (2006) The business–social policy nexus: corporate power and corporate inputs into social policy, *Journal of Social Policy*, 35(3): 473–494.

Fooks, G.J., Gilmore, A.B., Smith, K.E. et al. (2011) Corporate social responsibility and access to policy élites: an analysis of tobacco industry documents, *PLoS Medicine*, 8(8): e1001076.

Fooks, G.J., Smith, J., Lee, K. et al. (2017) Controlling corporate influence in health policy making? An assessment of the implementation of article 5.3 of the World Health Organization framework convention on tobacco control, *Globalization and Health*, 13(1): 1–20.

Gilmore, A.B. and Fooks, G. (2012) Global Fund needs to address conflict of interest, *Bulletin of the World Health Organization*, 90: 71–72.

Gleeson, D. and Labonté, R. (2020) *Trade Agreements and Public Health*. Singapore: Springer Nature.

Global Compact Office (2002) *The Global Compact: Report on Progress and Activities*. New York: United Nations.

Grüning, T., Weishaar, H., Collin, J. et al. (2012) Tobacco industry attempts to influence and use the German government to undermine the WHO Framework Convention on Tobacco Control, *Tobacco Control*, 21(1): 30–38.

Hanefeld, J., Hawkins, B., Knai, C. et al. (2016) What the InBev merger means for health in Africa, *BMJ Global Health*, 1: e000099.

Hawkins, B., and Holden, C. (2016) A corporate veto on health policy? Global constitutionalism and investor-state dispute settlement, *Journal of Health Politics, Policy and Law*, 41(5): 969–995.

Hawkins, B., Holden, C., Eckhardt, J. et al. (2018a) Reassessing policy paradigms: a comparison of the global tobacco and alcohol industries, *Global Public Health*, 13(1): 1–19.

Hawkins, B., Holden, C. and MacKinder, S. (2018b) A multi-level, multi-jurisdictional strategy: transnational tobacco companies' attempts to obstruct tobacco packaging restrictions, *Global Public Health*, 14(4): 570–583.

Hawkins, B. and McCambridge, J. (2020) Tied up in a legal mess: the alcohol industry's use of litigation to oppose minimum alcohol pricing in Scotland, *Scottish Affairs*, 29(1): 3–23.

Hawkins, B. and McCambridge, J. (2021) Alcohol policy, multi-level governance and corporate political strategy: the campaign for Scotland's minimum unit pricing in Edinburgh, London and Brussels, *The British Journal of Politics and International Relations*, 23(3): 391–409.

Holden, C. and Hawkins, B. (2018) Law, market building and public health in the European Union, *Global Social Policy*, 18(1): 45–61.

Hurt, R.D., Ebbert, J.O., Muggli, M.E. et al. (2009, May) Open doorway to truth: legacy of the Minnesota tobacco trial, *Mayo Clinic Proceedings*, 84(5): 446–456.

Jarman, H. (2013) Attack on Australia: tobacco industry challenges to plain packaging, *Journal of Public Health Policy*, 34(3): 375–387.

Jones, P.S. (2012) Powering up the people? The politics of indigenous rights implementation: International Labour Organisation Convention 169 and hydroelectric power in Nepal, *The International Journal of Human Rights*, 16(4): 624–647.

Lencucha, R. (2010) Philip Morris versus Uruguay: health governance challenged, *The Lancet*, 376(9744): 852–853.

Marten, R. and Hawkins, B. (2018) Stop the toasts: the Global Fund's disturbing new partnership, *The Lancet*, 391(10122): 735–736.

Matthes, B.K., Robertson, L. and Gilmore, A.B. (2020) Needs of LMIC-based tobacco control advocates to counter tobacco industry policy interference: insights from semi-structured interviews, *BMJ Open*, 10(11): e044710.

McCambridge, J., Hawkins, B. and Holden, C. (2013) Industry use of evidence to influence alcohol policy: a case study of submissions to the 2008 Scottish government consultation, *PLoS Medicine*, 10(4): e1001431.

McCambridge, J., Hawkins, B. and Holden, C. (2014) Vested interests in addiction research and policy. The challenge corporate lobbying poses to reducing society's alcohol problems: insights from UK evidence on minimum unit pricing, *Addiction*, 109(2): 199–205.

McCambridge, J., Mialon, M. and Hawkins, B. (2018) Alcohol industry involvement in policymaking: a systematic review, *Addiction*, 113(9): 1571–1584.

McKee, M. and Stuckler, D. (2018) Revisiting the corporate and commercial determinants of health, *American Journal of Public Health*, 108(9): 1167–1170.

Mialon, M. and McCambridge, J. (2018) Alcohol industry corporate social responsibility initiatives and harmful drinking: A systematic review, *The European Journal of Public Health*, 28(4): 664–673.

Moodie, R., Stuckler, D., Monteiro, C. et al. (2013) Profits and pandemics: prevention of harmful effects of tobacco, alcohol, and ultra-processed food and drink industries, *The Lancet*, 381(9867): 670–679.

Muggli, M.E., Hurt, R.D. and Repace, J. (2004) The tobacco industry's political efforts to derail the EPA report on ETS, *American Journal of Preventive Medicine*, 26(2): 167–177.

Peeters, S., Costa, H., Stuckler, D. et al. (2016) The revision of the 2014 European tobacco products directive: an analysis of the tobacco industry's attempts to 'break the health silo', *Tobacco Control*, 25(1): 108–117.

Ralston, R., Hill, S.E., Gomes, F.D.S. et al. (2021) Towards preventing and managing conflict of interest in nutrition policy? An analysis of submissions to a consultation on a draft WHO tool, *International Journal of Health Policy and Management*, 10(5): 255–265.

Sell, S.K. (2003) *Private Power, Public Law: The Globalization of Intellectual Property Rights*. Cambridge: Cambridge University Press.

Utting, P. (2002) The Global Compact and civil society: averting a collision course, *Development in Practice*, 12(5): 644–647.

Van Beeman, O. (2019) *Heineken in Africa: A Multinational Unleashed*. London: Hurst Publishers.

Waxman, H.A. (2004) Politics of international health in the Bush Administration, *Development*, 47(2): 24–28.

Non-governmental actors in global health

12

Neil Spicer

Overview

This chapter looks at three 'non-traditional' types of global health actors: global civil society organizations, philanthropic foundations, and global health partnerships and initiatives. Each type of actor is described and defined, and the chapter looks at some of their roles and ways in which they seek to influence global health issues. It then considers some of the important opportunities and challenges that non-governmental actors have brought to global health governance.

Learning objectives

After working through this chapter, you will be able to:

- Understand what is meant by the term global civil society, philanthropic foundations, and global health partnerships and initiatives.
- Describe the roles and assess the increasing significance to global health governance of these actors.
- Critically assess opportunities and challenges to global health governance stemming from these actors.

Key terms

Global civil society: Organizations, institutions, networks, individuals, ideas and values located between family, state and market, and operating beyond national societies, policies and economies.

Global health partnerships and initiatives: Entities for coordinating and financing programmes for health problems or diseases, research and development, donating drugs, vaccines or other products, strengthening health systems, campaigning and advocacy, technical assistance or health service and system support.

Philanthropic foundations: Non-profit, non-governmental actors possessing a fund of their own, managed by trustees and directors, and promoting public welfare that includes social, educational, charitable, religious or other activities.

Emerging actors in global health

Shifts in global health governance have brought opportunities and challenges. Substantial increases in development assistance for health, from US$5 billion in 1990 to US$40.6 billion in 2019 (IHME 2020), have occurred in parallel with a growth – some would say a proliferation – of global health actors. Indeed, Hoffman and Cole (2018) suggested the number increased from around 50 in 1960 to 203 in 2018.

From the 1990s on, new types of global health actors have emerged, and the importance of different actors has changed. As we saw in Chapter 10, 'traditional' actors, namely bilateral donors from high-income countries, and health-related multilaterals such as the World Health Organization, UNICEF and the World Bank, remain important and influential in global health. However, 'new' global actors are growing in number and are challenging the importance of these traditional actors. These include philanthropic foundations and other civil society organizations, not least the Bill and Melinda Gates Foundation (BMGF), global health partnerships and initiatives including the Global Fund (also discussed in Chapter 5 and Chapter 10), transnational pharmaceutical corporations and other private sector actors, intergovernmental organizations such as the African Union and European Union, and research and knowledge generation organizations including universities, consultancies and think tanks (Spicer et al. 2020). So-called 'south-south cooperation' is expanding, particularly the global influence of the five 'BRICS' economies of Brazil, Russia, India, China and South Africa. China's impact is particularly important, with its growing contributions to global health financing and influence on global institutions and agendas. Collectively, these new actors are said to contribute to global health by introducing substantial new financial resources, as well as harnessing flexibility, creative thinking and bringing new ways of working to bear in tackling persistent and emerging global health problems. However, they have exaggerated existing, and indeed introduced new, challenges to global health governance that we will look at later in this chapter.

Global civil society organizations

Civil society is usually defined as being constituted by those organizations and activities that fall outside the state and the private sector, and as having a wide variety of forms and roles. Gomez's (2018: 1) definition of civil society captures the diversity within the sector:

non-governmental actors that create and participate in formal organizations and informal movements with the goal of unifying, expressing, and deepening their normative beliefs and policy interests, while providing a platform from which to engage in public advocacy, collective mobilization, and pressures for issue awareness, policy reform and implementation.

Civil society embraces a multiplicity of actors, organizations and arrangements including, but not limited to: labour unions, faith-based groups, professional associations, academic and research institutions, think tanks, human rights networks, consumer rights coalitions, social movements, social and sports clubs, political parties, charities, environmental groups, professional associations, social enterprises, philanthropic foundations, clubs and even criminal organizations and networks (Gomez 2018; Greer et al. 2018). When we talk about civil society organizations (CSOs), we usually mean 'public interest' CSOs that aim to benefit the public, whether as a whole or particular groups, and often, but not necessarily, vulnerable or marginalized communities. But 'private interest' CSOs also exist that support the commercial interests of companies, such as by lobbying governments on behalf of pharmaceutical corporations, although it is not uncommon for them to hide their commercial agendas, thereby blurring boundaries between the public and private sectors (McCoy and Hilson 2009).

CSOs are not, of course, a new type of actor; neither is their influence on health and other policies in democratic countries such as the UK a new thing. What is new is the dramatic increase in the number of these organizations operating at the global level and influencing global health policies and issues – up from 1983 in the early twentieth century to an estimated 37,000 in 2000 (McCoy and Hilson 2009; United Nations Department of Economic and Social Affairs 2021). Hence, we often hear the term *global civil society* being used. Marchetti (2016: 78) captures the increasing importance and some of the roles of global civil society organizations:

> *The presence of civil society organisations in international affairs has become increasingly relevant. They have played a role in agenda setting, international law-making and diplomacy. Further, they have been involved in the implementation and monitoring of a number of crucial global issues. These range from trade to development and poverty reduction, from democratic governance to human rights, from peace to the environment, and from security to the information society.*

✎ Activity 12.1

Identify a way that the availability of the internet and social media has impacted positively on civil society and a way that the internet and social media have impacted negatively on civil society.

Feedback

There are positive and negative ways the internet and social media platforms are influencing global civil society. In terms of positive effects, these technologies are enabling the growth of informal, spontaneous, 'organic' civil society, whereby individuals with limited or no funding or backing from formal organizational structures can rapidly communicate ideas with global audiences. This helps individuals to generate and access information, enables the rapid mobilization of supporters around global campaigns and protests, the lobbying of politicians, government officials and corporations, and the seeking of crowdfunding.

But there are also negative effects. One is the emergence of diverse and sometimes contradictory information, including the spreading of misinformation relating to science, medicine and health: everything from discrediting Covid-19 and other vaccinations, to undermining water fluoridation and genetically modified food products, to promoting inappropriate homeopathic treatments for serious diseases.

Some of the problems stemming from globalization have prompted civil society organizations to act. Globalization has also enabled the emergence of a global civil society. Globalization has created and increased global health and social problems, many of which are beyond the control or interest of country governments, such as global climate change, global pandemics, stark differences between rich and poor, gender inequalities and human rights and social justice problems, to which CSOs have responded, in part because traditional global health actors have not been able or willing (Mathurapote and Putthasri 2018). Globalization also allows CSOs to operate at the global level because of easy access to the internet and social media technologies enabling more extensive and immediate communication, leading to the creation of 'transnational advocacy networks' working beyond national boundaries. Indeed, changing information and communication technologies have led commentators to distinguish between more traditional, 'organized' civil society and the dramatic growth of a much more informal and spontaneous 'organic' civil society taking the form of online groups, activists and commentators, social media communities and bloggers and vloggers that use the internet as a platform for sharing ideas and gaining influence (World Economic Forum 2013; VanDyck 2017; Cooper 2018).

The growth of global civil society has also been enabled by increases in donor funding channelled through CSOs as implementers of health programmes in low- and middle-income countries, although this very often takes the form of short-term, ad-hoc project-based funding and has pushed CSOs into service-related roles (VanDyck 2017). Nevertheless, patterns of funding continue to change; some donors have reduced CSO funding in favour of private sector partners, imposed increasing rigorous requirements to demonstrate impact and regularly shift priorities between different health issues and countries.

Some governments are also 'closing space' on civil society by restricting overseas funding to CSOs within their countries (see below). CSOs can therefore have a fragile existence and must increasingly seek diverse funding sources from philanthropists, social entrepreneurs and even through social investment products and crowdfunding (World Economic Forum 2013).

The roles and activities of CSOs are as diverse as the types of organizations. Greer et al. (2018) provide a framework to capture these major roles:

- **Policy activities:** these include engagement in, and attempts to influence and sometimes challenge, decision-making, such as advocacy, representing interests of different stakeholders, mobilizing broad public awareness and support, and holding powerful actors to account through generating and presenting evidence and engaging in watchdog activities.
- **Service activities:** providing a service, either to members of specific communities or to the general public.
- **Governance activities:** contributing to formulating technical standards, making and enforcing regulations and social partnership arrangements.

Global CSOs or international non-governmental organizations (INGOs) have used multiple mechanisms and approaches to successfully influence global health agendas, including: traditional lobbying; appealing to the media to take up their causes; publishing data and research, including in academic journals; posting material on the internet and through social media channels; participating in agency hearings, committees, debates and board meetings where they are invited to contribute, or using these platforms to lobby power decision-makers; and presenting at and participating in international conferences and workshops (Cooper 2018; Gomez 2018). Indeed, these organizations have influenced many important and contentious global health issues. For example, they played a key role in promoting breastfeeding by campaigning to establish an international code on the negative effects of infant formulas, known as the International Code for Marketing of Breast-milk Substitutes, and advocating for reduced tobacco consumption in low- and middle-income countries by contributing to the Framework Convention on Tobacco Control.

✎ Activity 12.2

Make a list of health issues civil society organizations have sought to influence at the global level in recent decades. Think of any health issues that you know of where CSOs have sought to have influence over policy.

Feedback

Civil society organizations have been involved in many health issues, including: universal access to healthcare; access to antiretroviral treatment and other medicines; gender-based violence; harm caused by alcohol and tobacco; abortion laws; genetically modified crops; mental health issues; Covid-19 vaccine access.

What is clear is that CSOs are increasingly shifting their stance from 'outsiders' targeting governments and other powerful health actors with policy activities, including advocacy campaigns, lobbying and acting as critical watchdogs, to 'insiders' partnering with other global health actors as members of governance mechanisms and networks (McCoy and Hilson 2009). For example, many CSOs contribute to global health by working with or being formally affiliated with UN agencies, although these agencies do not tend to allow formal representation of CSOs in decision-making (Gomez 2018). For example, the WHO invites CSOs to input at technical working groups and committees that it convenes at global, regional and country levels. CSOs also influence global health through participation in global health partnerships and initiatives, including the Global Fund and the GAVI Alliance (Global Alliance for Vaccines and Immunization) alongside governments, UN agencies and corporations. Indeed, their participation is increasingly formalized through having voting seats on decision-making boards, although some commentators suggest that this has increased corporations' influence on global health more than that of civil society and that northern country based international CSOs tend to be better represented in these groups and committees than smaller CSOs from low- and middle-income countries (see also Chapter 11). Indeed, civil society membership of Country Coordination Mechanisms within countries receiving Global Fund support, which is a requirement of the Fund, tends to be dominated by larger, better funded international CSOs than smaller grass roots community-based organizations, leading some to criticize this arrangement for being tokenistic (Gomez 2018; Spicer et al. 2011; Storeng and de Bengy Puyvallee 2018).

✏ **Activity 12.3**

Thinking about a country you are familiar with, identify both positive and negative ways that increasing access to funding from bilateral donors and global health partnerships and initiatives might change the role of civil society in global health policy.

Feedback

There are several ways in which increasing access to funding may strengthen civil society and its role in global health policy. In terms of positive effects, receiving donor funding may help CSOs to invest in management and financial systems, and this increasing professionalism can improve how governments and global actors perceive them. As recipients of Global Fund grants, CSOs can also be part of decision-making processes through Country Coordination Mechanisms and have better access to powerful actors, including government actors and development partners. Funding from bilateral donors and global health partnerships and initiatives can also enable them to travel to global meetings and conferences or obtain technologies that allow participation virtually in meetings, allowing them to have access to fora involved in global-level decisions and develop networks and alliances with other global actors.

There can also be more negative effects. Increasing dependence on funding from bilateral donors and global health partnerships and initiatives leads some commentators to accuse funders of co-opting CSOs, leading the latter to compromise their values and weaken ties with the communities and groups they claim to represent. This may also mute their voices as they shift away from more critical advocacy or watchdog roles towards service provision.

Philanthropic foundations

As Chapter 4 explored in historical context, philanthropic foundations are a particular form of civil society organization and can be defined as non-profit, non-governmental actors possessing a fund of their own, managed by trustees and directors and promoting public welfare, including social, educational, charitable, religious or other activities. However, it can be difficult to differentiate between foundations and other non-profit, non-governmental organizations, in part because the term is often used interchangeably with 'endowment', 'trust' or 'fund' and captures diverse types of actors that include private and public foundations, corporate foundations, single social entrepreneurs, venture philanthropists and, more recently, 'philanthrocapitalists' – a term coined by Bishop and Green to describe philanthropists adopting business approaches to philanthropy, and sometimes even conflating business aims with charitable work (Bishop and Green 2008).

When talking about philanthropic foundations and global health, we usually think of the BMGF, established in the 1990s, not least because of its substantial annual grants; in 2019 these totalled US$2.7 billion

(BMGF 2021). With a large contribution in 2006 from Warren Buffet, a US investor and philanthropist, worth over US$30 billion, and again in 2020 worth US$12.7 billion, it became the largest private donor to the WHO and the second largest donor overall after the US government. There are other well-known foundations, and many of the largest are from the USA, such as the Rockefeller Foundation (established 1913) and the Ford Foundation (established 1936) and from the UK, including the Carnegie Foundation (established 1905) and the Wellcome Trust (established 1936). Foundations from middle-income countries are also important, such as the Carlos Slim Foundation from Mexico established in 1986 and Tata Trusts from India, established in 1919. Indeed, many foundations are not new; neither is their ability to influence global health. The Rockefeller Foundation, for instance, played an important role in establishing the League of Nations Health Organization, including providing 40 per cent of the organization's original budget (see also the discussion in Chapter 4) (Birn and Fee 2013).

Among the advantages that foundations have over traditional bilateral and multilateral global health actors is their relative freedom to transfer innovative approaches from the business world to health and other development issues, as well as their dynamic and entrepreneurial spirit. They are often able to draw attention to issues that are not emphasized by traditional actors and can be freer than other actors to criticize governments and pressurize them to act (Reubi 2018). Large foundations have become important global health actors, with much of their influence stemming from their substantial contributions to increasing development assistance for health over recent decades. While philanthropic organizations are not always particularly transparent about their financing, estimates suggest that, overall, they donated US$12.6 billion for health work in low- and middle-income countries in the period 2013–2015, 72 per cent of which came from the BMGF (OECD 2019a). By the year 2019, private philanthropists including the BMGF, were contributing US$8.4 billion annually for development assistance for health, representing over 20 per cent of the US$40.6 billion total (IHME 2020).

The BMGF with its large contributions to the WHO and the Global Fund is widely credited with injecting energy into global health and increasing global attention on diseases such as malaria and polio, and more recently the BMGF has pledged very substantial funds for the global Covid-19 response, including the development of Covid-19 vaccines and their affordable access in low- and middle-income countries (Cheney 2020). It is also a key member and funder of a number of global partnerships and networks, including Roll Back Malaria and the Global Alliance for Improved Nutrition, and BMGF funding of US$750 million helped establish the GAVI Alliance in 2000. The BMGF was even a member of 'H8', an elite group of global health actors that included the World Bank and the health-related UN agencies, the GAVI Alliance and the Global

Fund, and was a signatory of the high-profile International Health Partnership global compact in 2007 (Buse and Harmer 2009; Tichenor and Sridhar 2018).

Global health partnerships and initiatives

Global health partnerships (GHPs), a term often used interchangeably with global public–private partnerships (GPPPs) and sometimes global health initiatives (GHIs), captures a range of financing, coordinating and implementing entities that are diverse in their functions, size and scope. Some focus on a specific health problem or disease, others on research and development of or donation of new drugs, vaccines or other products, or working on broader health systems issues, raising consciousness through campaigning and advocacy, technical assistance or health service and system support (Buse and Harmer 2009).

In the late 1990s and early 2000s, the urgent need to address persistent and newly emerging global health threats such as HIV/AIDS was increasingly acknowledged, and this meant that new thinking was required to harness the energy, business skills, innovative ideas and expertise, and financial resources of partnerships of both traditional and new actors – including civil society and foundations, as well as businesses such as pharmaceutical corporations (Walt et al. 2009). Hence, many global health partnerships and initiatives were created in the late 1990s and early 2000s and have become 'part of mainstream global health discourse and a dominant model for cooperation in a complex world' (Buse and Harmer 2009: 245). The WHO Maximizing Positive Synergies Collaborative Group (2009) listed around 100 GHPs and GHIs with involvement of several stakeholders covering health issues as diverse as HIV/AIDS, malaria, tuberculosis, vaccines, drugs for neglected tropical diseases, schistosomiasis, diarrhoea control, handwashing and reproductive health to name a few.

Some of the largest and best-known GHPs and GHIs include the Global Fund to Fight AIDS, Tuberculosis and Malaria (Global Fund), the GAVI Alliance and the President's Emergency Plan for AIDS Relief (PEPFAR). These and others have mobilized substantial additional funding for health programmes. Such funding equates to a considerable proportion of overall development aid for health in many low- and middle-income countries, and in some countries, external funding from GHPs and GHIs for HIV/AIDS exceeds domestic budgets for health as a whole. This has led to a dramatic scaling up of HIV/AIDS programmes and has improved access to services for populations with a limited ability to pay (Biesma et al. 2009; Walt et al. 2009).

GHPs and GHIs are also credited with raising the profile of certain health issues on national and international policy agendas, strengthening country

policy processes and health delivery capacity, and establishing international norms and standards. They have also brought some consensus
among different partners with diverse interests, although this consensus
has been delicate (Walt et al. 2009). For instance, there has been broad
agreement about the urgent need to mobilize substantial resources for
programmes to tackle HIV/AIDS, particularly in the countries of east and
southern Africa. However, differences between two of the biggest GHIs –
the Global Fund and PEPFAR – illustrate a lack of global agreement about
the best approach to doing this. The Global Fund, with its complex multi-
partner governance arrangements, finances recipient country proposals for
the three focal diseases and channels funds through a mix of government
and CSO implementers via a 'Principal Recipient'. PEPFAR, on the other
hand, is a bilateral HIV/AIDS programme of the US government that adopts
a more prescriptive approach and aims at rapid results by channelling the
bulk of its funding through mostly large, US-based CSO recipients. At
the time of its inception, there was also strong disagreement about what
the focus of the Global Fund should be; some actors called for a fund that
would address broad health systems strengthening issues in low- and
middle-income countries, while others pushed for a more targeted fund for
the rapid scale-up of interventions to tackle the three focal diseases. In the
end, those pushing for a more vertical approach won the argument,
although more recent Global Fund funding rounds accept country proposals
for health systems strengthening work (Ooms et al. 2007; Global Fund
2021).

Challenges: more actors = better health governance?

The explosion in the numbers of new global actors – 'a dazzling kaleido-
scopic environment' according to Walt et al. (2009) – creates important
challenges for global health actors and the countries receiving aid for
health. This section outlines some of the key challenges linked to this
change in the global health policy environment.

Harmonization and alignment

Fragmentation has become a major problem: that is, poor coordination
among different global health actors and implementers ('harmonization')
and between externally funded health programmes and recipient government policies, programmes, systems and targets ('alignment'). Spicer et
al. (2020) point to five interconnected causes of fragmentation among
global health actors:

1. **Proliferation of global health actors:** the very substantial increase in
   the number and types of global health actors has made effective coordination more and more challenging.

2. **Problems of global leadership:** the WHO's role as lead coordinator in global health is made difficult by the proliferation of global health actors and has been undermined by pressure from donors with divergent agendas and expectations.

3. **Divergent interests:** global health actors' interests are diverse, and their efforts in global health are commonly driven by self-interest, such as health security (protecting their own populations from the threat of communicable diseases) and foreign policy and economic interests; these interests are usually best served through less coordinated approaches such as 'vertical' health programmes and projects.

4. **Problems of accountability:** global health actors' weak accountability to low- and middle-income countries undermines alignment of health programmes to country priorities and policies, and strong accountability to high-income donor countries that fund them undermines the harmonization of the multitude of global health programmes.

5. **Problems of power relations:** global health financing and institutions are dominated by high-income countries and their interests, making it difficult for many low- and middle-income countries to influence global health actors' priorities and coordinate multiple health programmes within their countries.

Poor harmonization and alignment often have damaging effects on recipient countries with fragile health systems. This has been an enduring feature of the global health landscape and is arguably getting worse as the number of global health actors increases (Spicer et al. 2020). Donors, including GHPs and GHIs, often introduce parallel monitoring and evaluation and financial management procedures and duplicate coordination mechanisms, adding to already complex governance arrangements that place a considerable burden on recipient country governments. Like many bilateral health programmes before them, many of the GHPs and GHIs have introduced 'vertical', health issue-specific programmes and projects focused on single illnesses or topics, rather than broad, 'horizontal' primary healthcare interventions, which are criticized for imposing external priorities on recipient countries leading to a skewing of national policies and reducing 'country ownership' – the power and influence of recipient governments to determine their own policies and priorities (Biesma et al. 2009; Gostin and Mok 2009; WHO Maximizing Positive Synergies Collaborative Group 2009; Frenk and Moon 2013; Spicer et al. 2020). Sridhar (2010: 6) captures these issues:

> . . . lack of alignment of donors with the national approach, lack of harmonization among donors, and excessive transaction costs on recipient governments. Too often donors have their own ways of implementing initiatives in a country, thereby weakening national health strategies and systems . . .

Multiple high-profile declarations and initiatives signal global recognition of the problems of aid effectiveness, including the Paris Declaration of Aid Effectiveness (from 2005), followed by the International Health Partnership *Plus* (from 2007), both of which proposed principles of more predictable, longer-term aid commitments, improved harmonization and alignment, and better government ownership of externally funded programmes. Such high-profile initiatives remain an important part of the global health landscape. For example, a key initiative launched in 2019 was the Global Action Plan: Stronger Collaboration, Better Health (from 2019) that has been depicted as an important step forward towards better coordination among multilateral health organizations, and thereby helping to achieve the health-related SDGs. In 2021 there are calls for an international treaty for pandemic preparedness and prevention to promote global approaches to tackling Covid-19 and future pandemics. Shorten et al. (2012) listed no fewer than 19 major aid effectiveness declarations, initiatives and processes since the 1980s demonstrating sustained global resolve but also revealing that despite these efforts, the problems of aid effectiveness do not appear to be diminishing. This raises questions about whether global commitments have been effective and are reflected in improved practices on the ground. Spicer et al. (2020) suggested that the proliferation of such efforts to improve coordination has added to complexity of the global health architecture, and hence ironically, this has worsened the problems of coordination. Moreover, the voluntary and non-binding nature of most of these initiatives, with weak or absent accountability mechanisms in the event of failure to follow through on commitments, has limited their impacts.

Accountability and legitimacy

While many commentators welcome the shifts in power and influence the growth of civil society represents, this uncoordinated 'swarm' of global CSOs is viewed by some as a potential threat to the dominance of governments, UN agencies and transnational corporations. One criticism relates to whether CSOs are accountable in the same way as country governments are to voters, citizens and taxpayers, and the extent to which they are democratic. Civil society tends to be stronger in countries that are more democratic than those that are less democratic, and the existence of civil society can strengthen democracy through its ability to challenge and hold powerful governments, and indeed transnational corporations and multilateral agencies, to account. However, unlike (many) national governments, CSOs are not democratically elected: they do not represent populations in the same ways as elected governments of countries do. Some commentators point to parallels between donor-funded international and northern country-based CSOs and colonial administrators and missionaries imposing ideas and values on low- and middle-income country governments (Doyle and Patel 2008). Indeed, while funding from donors and foundations may empower and enable CSOs to act at the global level, this may at the same time weaken links to, and ability to benefit, the vulnerable and marginalized groups they claim to represent – and hence lines of accountability may be stronger 'upwards' to funders than 'downwards' to those communities (Green 2017). With very substantial global funding channelled through CSO health programme implementers, and thereby bypassing governments of low- and middle-income countries, the ability of the latter to build and maintain democratic legitimacy may be undermined (Doyle and Patel 2008; McCoy and Hilson 2009; Spicer et al. 2011; Green 2017; Cooper 2018).

Some commentators suggest that the problems of a lack of accountability and legitimacy may be particularly problematic in the case of some of the largest foundations, such as the BMGF, which have substantial power to influence decisions at global and country level derived from their huge resources. At the same time, they lack the formal public accountability mechanisms of most governments and UN agencies. While the BMGF is widely credited with energizing and raising the profile of global health issues, critics have pointed to its lack of transparency and limited involvement of other actors in its decision-making, poor alignment of its grant-making with country health priorities, and the fact that it tends to channel the bulk of its funding through US and other high-income country-based CSO implementers, thereby side-lining smaller CSOs from low- and middle-income countries and recipient governments (McGoey 2008; McGoey 2015; Reubi 2018; Tichenor and Sridhar 2018; Youde 2019).

Foundations have also been criticized for potential conflicts of interest. Among some of the larger foundations there are significant investments in pharmaceutical and food corporations, overlapping board directorships with these corporations and examples of partnership arrangements where corporations potentially benefit from foundations' tax-exempt status. The BMGF is a major shareholder of the Coca-Cola Corporation, which it has supported to develop new supply chains. Critics argue that while there are clear links between consumption of sugary drinks and rises in diabetes and obesity (which are overtaking infectious diseases as the major source of ill health in many low- and middle-income countries), the BMGF's investments in non-communicable diseases have been low (Stuckler et al. 2011; Elias et al. 2018). There have been calls for foundations to improve accountability and transparency, to focus investments on strengthening health systems rather than commodities and technologies, and to place more emphasis than they currently do on important global health issues prioritized by scientific evidence (Stuckler et al. 2011; McGoey 2015; Reubi 2018; Youde 2019).

Power and money

As well as being heterogeneous in their type and roles, CSOs are very diverse in size. Well-known northern CSOs such as Médecins sans

Frontières, Oxfam and Save the Children are highly professionalized and well resourced in contrast to the multitude of smaller CSOs, especially those based in low- and middle-income countries. As well as far greater capacity and resources, the former have far better access to and influence at the global level than the latter. Indeed, many smaller, low- and middle-income-based CSOs lack the capacity and resources to engage in global-level discussions, which often involve attending meetings in Geneva or Washington – although, as Chapter 3 discussed, the internet and social media may be changing this (Cooper 2018). Certainly, in terms of funding health and other development work, donor country-based and international CSOs dominate. By 2017, less than 7 per cent of all official development assistance channelled to and through CSOs went to low- and middle-income country-based CSOs; most of the remainder was channelled through international CSOs and/or CSOs from the donor countries (OECD 2019b). However, the ability (and legitimacy) of these large, well-funded northern CSOs to represent the views and needs of poor, marginalized groups in low- and middle-income countries has been questioned: some commentators suggest they are more in tune with dominant ideas about globalization and global health, and potentially the economic interests of donor countries, than potentially more critical ideas and perspectives of marginalized groups (Doyle and Patel 2008; McCoy and Hilson 2009; Green 2017; Cooper 2018; Spicer et al. 2020).

Another concern relates to the potential for co-option of CSOs by bilateral donors, foundations and other global funders, resulting in shifts away from political activities including more critical advocacy or watchdog roles to service activities, involving dependency of CSOs on funding to implement health programmes – thereby, tending to serve the interests of powerful global health actors, while attenuating CSOs' ability to challenge those actors. This may have professionalized some low- and middle-income country-based CSOs, which, for example, have adopted stronger monitoring and evaluation and financial management systems in accordance with donor requirements, and hence enabled them to work effectively alongside government and development partners. However, adopting more grant-driven business models, often based on short-term project funding, can also mute CSOs' ability to challenge and hold governments, donors and other powerful actors to account on controversial issues such as drug use, sex work and HIV/AIDS – and thereby bring about transformative social change (Doyle and Patel 2008; Spicer et al. 2011; Harmer et al. 2013; Green 2017). Donors' requirements for quantifiable results have also tended to shift the attention of CSOs towards activities that are more measurable and easily achievable in the short term, rather than longer-term or systemic changes. Moreover, CSOs' dependence on ad-hoc project funding, preoccupies their efforts on seeking future funding rather than gaining buy-in from communities and ensuring their work is sustainable (Cooper 2018; Green 2017). As Spicer et al. (2011) note, based on a study in three former Soviet Union countries:

'[The Global Fund] turned the civil society sector into robots just implementing donors' ideas'. This led to heightened competition among CSO implementers for finite donor funding, thereby undermining civil society collective action, and by bypassing country governments in favour of civil society, donors undermined country ownership and created tensions between government and civil society (Spicer et al. 2011; Harmer et al. 2013). In Chapter 6, we also explore how commercial sector actors work with and sometimes co-opt CSOs.

Some CSOs are also under pressure from their own country governments, which are 'closing space', that is creating increasingly difficult and restricted operating environments for CSOs, particularly for those advocating for improved human rights and democratic principles and practices. The governments of Zimbabwe, Ethiopia, Russia, Hungary and many other countries have adopted a range of approaches to closing spaces such as increased surveillance of CSO activities through intercepting mobile phone messages, imposing media restrictions, shutting down the internet and social media platforms, restricting legal and regulatory rules around international donor funding, and sometimes through harassment, detention, smear campaigns and even violence (World Economic Forum 2013; Kreienkamp 2017; Cooper 2018).

Summary

In this chapter, you have learnt about the diversity of CSOs, philanthropic foundations and global health partnerships and initiatives, and assessed the increasing significance of these 'new' actors in decision-making at the global level. You also critically appraised some key challenges: problems of coordinating the increasing numbers of global health actors; problems of CSOs and foundations maintaining accountability and legitimacy; and the imbalances between large northern and small southern CSOs in terms of their influence on global health decisions.

References

Biesma, R., Brugha, R., Harmer, A. et al. (2009) The effects of global HIV/AIDS initiatives on country health systems: a review of the evidence, *Health Policy and Planning*, 24(4): 239–252.

Birn, A. and Fee, E. (2013) The Rockefeller Foundation and the international health agenda, *The Lancet*, 381(9878): 1618–1619.

Bishop, M. and Green, M. (2008) *Philanthrocapitalism: How the Rich can Save the World*. London: Bloomsbury Press.

BMGF (2021) Factsheet. Available at: https://globalization.gatesfoundation.org/Who-We-Are/General-Information/Foundation-Factsheet#:~:text=July%2017%2C%202017%3A%20%242.4%20billion,July%201%2C%202019%3A%20%242.7%20billion (accessed 21 May 2021).

Buse, K. and Harmer, A. (2009) Global health partnerships: the mosh pit of global health governance, in K. Buse, W. Hein and N. Drager (eds) *Making Sense of Global Health Governance: A Policy Perspective*. Basingstoke: Palgrave Macmillan.

Cheney, C. (2020) Gates Foundation Covid-19 commitment reaches $1.75B with latest pledge, Devex. Available at: https://globalization.devex.com/news/gates-foundation-Covid-19-commitment-reaches-1-75b-with-latest-pledge-98739#:~:text=The%20Gates%20Foundation%20announced%20Wednesday,tests%2C%20vaccines%2C%20and%20treatments (accessed 21 May 2021).

Cooper, R. (2018) *What Is Civil Society? How Is the Term Used and What Is Seen to Be Its Role and Value (Internationally) in 2018? K4D Helpdesk Report.* Brighton, UK: Institute of Development Studies.

Doyle, C. and Patel, P. (2008) Civil society organizations and global health initiatives: problems of legitimacy, *Social Science and Medicine*, 66: 1928–1938.

Elias, C., Voorhies, R. and Mundel, T. (2018) Opinion: the global development community asks tough questions. Here are the answers, Devex. Available at: https://globalization.devex.com/news/opinion-the-global-development-community-asks-tough-questions-here-are-the-answers-92135 (accessed 21 May 2021).

Frenk, J. and Moon, S. (2013) Governance challenges in global health, *New England Journal of Medicine*, 368: 936–942.

Global Fund (2021) Resilient and sustainable systems for health. Available at: https://globalization.theglobalfund.org/en/resilient-sustainable-systems-for-health/ (accessed 20 June 2021).

Gomez, E. (2018) Civil society in global health policymaking: a critical review, *Globalization and Health*, 14: 73.

Gostin, L. and Mok, E. (2009) Grand challenges in global health governance, *British Medical Bulletin*, 90: 7–18.

Green, S. (2017) *Civil Society at a Crossroads: Exploring Sustainable Operating Models.* Washington, DC: Centre for Strategic and International Studies.

Greer, S., Wismar, M., Pastorino, G. et al. (2018) *Civil Society and Health: Contributions and Potential.* European Observatory on Health Systems and Policies.

Harmer, A., Spicer, N., Bogdan, D. et al. (2013) Has Global Fund support of civil society advocacy in the former Soviet Union established meaningful engagement or 'a lot of jabber about nothing'?, *Health Policy and Planning*, 28(3): 299–308.

Hoffman, S. and Cole, C. (2018) Defining the global health system and systematically mapping its network of actors, *Globalization and Health*, 14: 38.

IHME (2020) *Financing Global Health 2019: Tracking Health Spending in a Time of Crisis.* Seattle, WA: Institute for Health Metrics and Evaluation.

Kreienkamp, J. (2017) *Responding to the Global Crackdown on Civil Society.* London: Global Governance Unit, UCL.

Marchetti, R. (2016) Global civil society, in S. McGlinchey (ed.) *International Relations.* Bristol: E-International Relations Publishing.

Mathurapote, N. and Putthasri, W. (2018) The rise of civil society, *British Medical Journal*, 363: 14–15.

McCoy, D. and Hilson, M. (2009) Civil society, its organizations, and global health governance, in K. Buse, W. Hein and N. Drager (eds.) *Making Sense of Global Health Governance: A Policy Perspective.* Basingstoke: Palgrave Macmillan.

McGoey, L. (2008) Philanthrocapitalism and its critics, *Poetics*, 40: 185–199.

McGoey, L. (2015) *No Such Thing as a Free Gift: The Gates Foundation and the Price of Philanthropy.* London: Verso Books.

OECD (2019a) *Health and Philanthropy: Harnessing Novel Approaches for Improved Access to Quality Healthcare.* Available at: https://globalization.oecd.org/development/networks/2019_Health_policy_note.pdf (accessed 20 June 2021).

OECD (2019b) *Aid for Civil Society Organisations: Statistics Based on DAC Members' Reporting to the Creditor Reporting System Database, 2016–2017.* Available at: https://globalization.oecd.org/dac/financing-sustainable-development/development-finance-topics/Aid-for-CSOs-2019.pdf (accessed 20 June 2021).

Ooms, G., Van Damme, W. and Temmerman, M. (2007) Medicines without doctors: Why the global fund must fund salaries of health workers to expand AIDS treatment, *PLoS Medicine*, 4: 605–608.

Reubi, D. (2018) Epidemiological accountability: philanthropists, global health and the audit of saving lives, *Economy and Society*, 47(1): 83–110.

Shorten, T., Taylor, M., Spicer, N. et al. (2012) The *International Health Partnership Plus*: rhetoric or real change? Results of a self-reported survey in the run-up to the 4th High Level Forum on Aid Effectiveness in Busan, *Globalization and Health*, 8: 13.

Spicer, N., Agyepong, I., Ottersen, T. et al. (2020) 'It's far too complicated': why fragmentation persists in global health, *Globalization and Health*, 16: 60.

Spicer, N., Harmer, A., Bogdan, D. et al. (2011) Circus monkeys or change agents? Civil society advocacy for HIV/AIDS in adverse policy environments, *Social Science and Medicine*, 73(12): 1748–1755.

Sridhar, D. (2010) Seven challenges in international development assistance for health and ways forward, *Journal of Law, Medicine and Ethics*, 38(3): 459–469.

Storeng, K. and de Bengy Puyvallee, A. (2018) Civil society participation in global public private partnerships for health, *Health Policy and Planning*, 33: 928–936.

Stuckler, D., Basu, S. and McKee, M. (2011) Global health philanthropy and institutional relationships: how should conflicts of interest be addressed?, *PLoS Medicine*, 8(4): e1001020.

Tichenor, M. and Sridhar, D. (2018) Global health disruptors: the Bill and Melinda Gates Foundation, *British Medical Journal Opinion*, 28 November.

VanDyck, C. (2017) *Concept and Definition of Civil Society Sustainability*. Washington DC: Centre for Strategic and International Studies.

United Nations Department of Economic and Social Affairs (2021) NGO branch. Available at: http://csonet.org/index.php?menu=14 (accessed 20 June 2021).

Walt, G., Spicer, N. and Buse, K. (2009) Mapping the global health architecture, in K. Buse, W. Hein and N. Drager (eds.) *Making Sense of Global Health Governance: A Policy Perspective*. Basingstoke: Palgrave Macmillan.

World Economic Forum (2013) *The Future Role of Civil Society*. Geneva: World Economic Forum in collaboration with KPMG International.

World Health Organization Maximizing Positive Synergies Collaborative Group (2009) An assessment of interactions between global health initiatives and country health systems, *The Lancet*, 373 (9681): 2137–2169.

Youde, J. (2019) The role of philanthropy in international relations, *Review of International Studies*, 45(1): 39–56.

13

Trade and global health

Benjamin Hawkins

Overview

This chapter examines the global trade regime, including the role of the World Trade Organization (WTO) and its effects on global health. In addition, it focuses on the increasing number of bilateral and regional trade agreements (BRTIAs) that have become increasingly important components of the international trade system. This chapter builds on Chapter 2 on the global economy, Chapter 10 on bilateral and multilateral actors and Chapter 11 on the commercial sector.

Learning objectives

After working through this chapter, you will be able to:

- Describe the structure and functions of the WTO, and the WTO Agreement on Trade Related Aspects of Intellectual Property (TRIPS) and General Agreement on Trade in Services (GATS).
- Compare and contrast multilateral, regional and bilateral trade agreements.
- Critically assess the implications of the global trade regime for global health.

Key terms

Tariff: An import levy placed on imported goods, designed to make imports more expensive and thus protect domestic producers from overseas competition.

Non-tariff barrier: Barriers to trade that have an equivalent effect to tariffs. These may be quotas or quantitative restrictions on imports designed to protect domestic industries. They may also be internal taxes, administrative procedures and regulations that have trade-restrictive effects.

Investor-State Dispute Settlement (ISDS): A mechanism included in bilateral and regional trade agreements whereby private, commercial actors

(companies) can bring legal challenges directly against states whose policies and actions they believe infringe their rights as investors. This differs
from the WTO dispute resolution mechanism, whereby only member states
can bring cases against other states.

Trade liberalization and health

Economic theory suggests that international trade should lead to increased
economic growth, lower costs and wider access to goods and services for
consumers. In principle, therefore, increases in trade should lead to aggre-
gate increases in wealth through the more efficient allocation of resources
and the specialization of national economies on the sectors in which they
are most efficient or have a 'comparative advantage'. However, there are
often huge disparities in the distribution of the economic gains from trade
both within and between states (see Chapter 2 and Chapter 9). Trade liberalization – i.e. the reduction of barriers to trade as a result of bilateral,
regional and global trade agreements – can affect health in multiple ways.

Notwithstanding the distributional disparities of the benefits of trade
within and between states, increased economic growth and the greater
wealth of societies is associated with improved health outcomes at least in
the initial phases of economic development (Lange and Vollmer 2017).
However, there are numerous other ways in which trade impacts on health,
both positively and negatively, for example when a disease crosses borders together with a traded good or with individuals moving to deliver or
receive health services, or where a reduction in tariffs leads to greater
availability and lower purchase costs for medical equipment and devices.
Elsewhere, liberalization of trade in services that allows doctors and nurses
to practise across borders or to move from one country to another may
benefit the health system in their 'host' country through increases in
capacity but may have more negative effects on the health systems in
their country of origin, with implications for the cost, availability and quality
of health services for the local population. The signing of trade agreements
may also increase the availability and promotion of health-harming products such as tobacco, alcohol and processed foods associated with the
increased prevalence of non-communicable diseases (NCDs).

Trade agreements also have implications for health policy and regulatory
capacity at the national level. The inclusion of regulatory cooperation
clauses and dispute resolution mechanisms in trade agreements may
restrict domestic policymaking space and have implications for national
sovereignty by creating requirements for national policies to comply with
the commitments made by states in international agreements and creating
means by which other states and, at times, even corporations can challenge non-compliant laws.

The global trade regime – and the risks associated with cross-border movements of goods and service provision – creates particular demands on the governments and health systems of low- and middle-income countries (LMICs). As well as the need to regulate effectively to counter potential threats, these agreements may also restrict access to affordable pharmaceuticals (Gleeson et al. 2019). Furthermore, the negotiation, monitoring and management of trade agreements is expensive, skills-intensive and requires considerable infrastructure and staffing (e.g. in permanent delegations to the WTO in Geneva), with small and particularly poorer states at a considerable disadvantage in defending their interests and achieving their objectives (Jawara and Kwa 2004).

✎ Activity 13.1

Identify some goods that might have implications for public health if traded from one country to another. Describe what potential benefits and what risk might emerge from these arrangements. Think about potential health risks that may arise from the time a good arrives in the country, to their purchase and use by the end consumer. What are some of the practical considerations that national government and trade agreements might need to take into account in seeking to regulate this trade?

Feedback

Some examples of dangerous goods include tobacco products, contaminated foodstuffs, toxic chemicals and military weapons. Governments will need to include border inspection regimes (especially for food or products of animal and plant origin) to ensure that imports meet domestic health and safety standards. In addition, the entry of new brands and economic actors in a market may increase competition, advertising, marketing and competitive pricing which drive sales and thus harms. Consequently, governments may need to consider the secondary policy implications of a liberalization of trade in products such as alcohol. This may be minimum pricing to stop discounting or regulation of advertising.

The multilateral trade regime and the World Trade Organization

From 1947 to 1995 the rules of the multilateral trade regime were governed by the General Agreement on Tariffs and Trade (GATT), which became the driving force behind global trade liberalization over the 50 years following its foundation. It served as the forum for negotiating reductions in tariffs on traded goods through a series of 'trade rounds' held between

1947 and 1994. Tariffs fell on average from around 40 per cent in 1940 to 4 per cent in 1995 (Trading Economics 2013) and, on manufactured goods traded between advanced industrial economies, are now very low. Those on agricultural goods, meanwhile, remain much higher. The 'Uruguay Round' of GATT negotiations (1986–1994) resulted in the formation of the World Trade Organization (WTO) in January 1995. Under the WTO, trade rules expanded from a focus on goods and tariffs to cover other areas such as services and intellectual property rights, discussed in the sections below.

Based in Geneva, the WTO's governance structure is headed by a Director General. As a member-led organization, its top-level decision-making body is the Ministerial Conference, which brings together trade officials and ministers from member states at least once every two years. Below that sits the General Council, which meets several times a year and is attended by ambassadors and representatives from members' permanent trade delegations in Geneva. The General Council also undertakes regular reviews of WTO member states' national trade policies when it sits as the Trade Policy Review Body and, as will be discussed below, serves as the main arbitrary body in the dispute resolution process. The principles underpinning the world trading system under the WTO are:

* Non-discrimination
* Binding commitments
* Reciprocity
* Negotiated liberalization
* Transparency

WTO member states produce schedules of 'commitments' – essentially lists of the tariffs and quotas they will apply to each good and service they import – that they submit to the WTO secretariat. These binding commitments, along with the norm of transparency, are designed to create predictability and stability in the global trade regime. The principle of non-discrimination has two components: the 'most favoured nation' (MFN) principle and 'national treatment'. The former means that member states must offer the same concessions (e.g. tariff reductions) to all member states, so that no one country is treated more or less favourably than others. This relates also to the idea of reciprocity where concessions made by one state should be reciprocated. Similarly, if any member states are discriminated against by another member state they can take retaliatory measures having equal effect on trade. The principle of national treatment, meanwhile, means that WTO member states must treat overseas producers and suppliers no less favourably than domestic operators.

Trade in services

The establishment of the WTO also saw the creation of the General Agreement on Trade in Services (GATS), reflecting the ways in which services trade has been facilitated by new communications technologies and the increasing access to, and affordability of, international travel. GATS defines four modes of service delivery:

- **Mode 1: cross-border supply**. The provision of services in one country by suppliers in another country, e.g. remote diagnosis or treatment planning (i.e. e-medicine).
- **Mode 2: consumption abroad**. The movement of consumers from one country to another in order to receive services in that country (i.e. 'medical tourism').
- **Mode 3: commercial presence**. The establishment of service provision facilities overseas (i.e. 'foreign direct investment').
- **Mode 4: presence of natural persons.** Service provision by individuals in another country (i.e. the movement of doctors, nurses and other health professionals overseas).

Recent decades have seen a growth in almost all of these modes of provision in relation to trade in health services, and the increasing trade in services has important implications for patient health and health systems.

Health exceptions under WTO law

WTO law specifically recognizes health protections and the need in certain circumstances to restrict trade to protect public health. Under certain conditions, member states may restrict trade on goods under Article XX GATT (with similar provisions set out for services in Article XVI GATS) in order to protect the health of humans, animals and plants on the condition that the restriction is non-discriminatory (i.e. applies to all states), is scientifically justified and it can be established that the same outcomes could not have been achieved through less trade-restrictive measures. These requirements are designed to ensure that such mechanisms are not used as a disguised form of protectionism and such measures may give rise to disputes (see below) if other member states feel their goods or service providers are being unfairly excluded from a national market on spurious health grounds.

The logic of the WTO is to move towards ever greater trade liberalization through periodic rounds of negotiations between its member states. However, the formal principle of multilateralism must be viewed in the context of the huge asymmetries of power between WTO member states. This means that while all states have the same formal decision-making power within the WTO, its agreements reflect the interests of the largest economies: the USA, the European Union (EU), Japan and, in recent decades, China. The latest round of WTO negotiations – the Doha Round, launched in 2001 and targeting further trade liberalization and integration of LMICs into global trade – stalled soon after its inception and has made little progress towards an agreement, due principally to disputes between high-income countries and LMICs relating to a range of issues including agricultural subsidies and protections for food producers in high-income countries. Without these subsidies, farmers in the USA and the EU, for example, would be far less competitive than producers from LMICs.

✎ **Activity 13.2**

In recent decades there has been substantial movement of health professionals (e.g. doctors and nurses) across borders to work in health systems overseas. At the same time there has been an increasing propensity for patients to seek treatment overseas. What are the implications of this for the health systems in the home and destination countries of health professionals and patients? What are the potential risks and benefits from this trade in services?

Feedback

In terms of the movement of doctors and nurses overseas:

- The destination country would need to ensure that they can verify professional qualifications and that these are of an equivalent scope and standard to those domestically.
- There may be language and other cultural factors affecting communications and thus effective diagnosis and treatment, between practitioners and patients.
- The country of origin of medical practitioners overseas may suffer from a 'brain drain' as a result of which they lack sufficient doctors and nurses for local service provision.
- The costs of training medical professionals would thus fall on (mainly low-income) exporter countries, while other (mainly high-income) counties would reap the benefit of this through their work there.

In terms of receiving medical services overseas, the key issues to consider include:

- Identifying a qualified, reliable doctor and other medical service providers and understanding the regulatory regimes in place to ensure the quality of treatment.
- Potential language barriers and communications issues, as well as cultural differences and specificities.
- How the service would be paid for, including costs arising from any unforeseen medical complications not predicted in advance.

- From a systems perspective, there are potential costs and additional pressures that may be placed on the health system in the patient's home state. For example, on returning home from non-essential surgery overseas you may need ongoing secondary care and medical treatment, which creates a cost on their domestic health system and government finances.
- Finally, 'medical tourism' may divert resources away from health services for local populations in the destination country.

The WTO dispute resolution process

An important innovation of the WTO was the creation of a new procedure for settling trade disputes: the WTO Dispute Settlement Body (DSB). It is important to note that only member states have the standing to bring cases to the DSB, and these deal only with issues relating to non-compliance with WTO agreements or commitments. Private entities (e.g. companies or trade unions) and individuals adversely affected by trade issues cannot complain directly to the WTO but can lobby member states to bring cases that affect their interests. Powerful corporations, often with close association with the governments in their home states, may have significant capacity to induce governments to bring cases in their interests. Since they are important sources of employment and tax revenue, governments are keen to defend the interests of important national companies or multinationals based in their territory.

When a dispute is lodged, a panel of experts is established by the DSB to consider the case and has the sole authority to accept or reject the panel's findings and, where complaints are upheld, will set out what measures are necessary to bring that state back into compliance with their WTO obligations. Parties to a dispute settlement case have recourse to appeal the judgment in front of a specialist Appellate Body. Following the outcome of a dispute resolution process, the WTO has the power to authorize compensation or the retaliatory suspension of concessions by the plaintiff state, if the offending country fails to comply with a DSB ruling.

The TRIPS agreement and access to medicines

The TRIPS agreement, enacted by the WTO at its inception in 1995, sets out minimum standards for protecting and enforcing nearly all forms of intellectual property (IP) rights (i.e. patents, trademarks and copyright), which has obvious implications for global health. All WTO member states must comply with these standards, where necessary modifying their national legislation to bring it into line with their commitments under TRIPS. However, Article 8 of the agreement explicitly acknowledges that, in framing national laws, members may 'adopt measures necessary to protect public health and nutrition, and to promote the public interest'.

Under TRIPS, pharmaceutical products are accorded full intellectual property rights (IPR), meaning that these companies could prevent others from producing or using new products. The strength of the IP provisions in the WTO agreement – indeed the inclusions of IP provisions in the agreement at all – reflects the role played by industry actors in lobbying for their inclusion via the United States Trade Representative (Sell 2003). The pharmaceutical industry argues that such rights reflect the very high research and development costs and the absence of such protections would undermine new treatments coming to market. However, this is contested by many global health actors who highlight the vital role played by public funding and public private collaborations (e.g. with public universities) and the relatively high percentage of non-research costs accrued by drug companies (e.g. on marketing) (see Light and Warburton 2011).

Within the global health community, TRIPS raises concerns about access to medicines, particularly in LMIC settings via the production of less expensive generic medicines. In 2001 the South African government sought an amendment to the South African Medicines and Related Substances Control Amendment Act that would allow the import and use of cheaper generic versions of prescription drugs, including anti-retroviral drugs (ARVs) needed to help tackle the country's HIV/AIDS epidemic. The government undertook to 'parallel import' the cheapest drug available and granted 'compulsory licensing' allowing companies to make copies of patented drugs without the owners' permission. The government argued that the rapidly rising prevalence of HIV/AIDS in the country constituted a public health emergency justifying such measures under the health derogations set out in the TRIPS agreement. Global pharmaceutical companies, including GlaxoSmithKline, Merck and Roche launched legal action in 1998 but dropped the case in April 2001. Following this, the 2001 WTO Ministerial Conference in Qatar issued the so-called 'Doha Declaration' acknowledging the ability of WTO members to protect public health and promote access to medicines through compulsory licences parallel imports, albeit with some restrictions (Correa 2004). However, since the Doha Declaration, some countries including the USA and the EU – in which the largest pharmaceutical companies are based – have included so-called 'TRIPS Plus' IP protections into trade agreements they have concluded with other states (Sell 2007).

Bilateral and regional trade and investment agreements

The consequence of the lack of progress in the Doha round of WTO negotiations launched in 2001 has been a proliferation of bilateral and regional trade and investment agreements (BRTIAs) concluded between states with the purpose of trade liberalization outside the WTO system. These types of agreements have always been part of the multilateral trade regime, and indeed WTO law makes explicit provision for these, allowing for derogations from core WTO principles (such as the MFN principle) for the parties to such agreements. Consequently, it is possible for states to agree zero tariffs on certain goods within a bilateral or regional trade agreement while still applying higher tariff rates to WTO member states with whom they have no such agreements. In addition, the proliferation of regional trade agreements reflects the fact that countries tend to trade most extensively and intensively with those closest to them (the so-called 'gravity model' of trade), which creates a rationale for codifying and normalizing trading relations with your closest neighbours through such accords (De Benedictis and Taglioni 2011).

BRTIAs have served as a mechanism through which the most economically powerful states have sought to promote their trade interests beyond what has been possible for them to achieve within the WTO, for example including more robust IP measures to protect patented drug producers in their territory. While the WTO has been criticized extensively for favouring the interests of the Global North over the Global South, the power dynamics involved in bilateral and inter-regional negotiations are perhaps even starker than those present in multilateral forums. When entering into negotiations with a single other state, or small group of states, there is less possibility of poorer nations pooling their resources and acting collectively – as they have done with the G90 grouping at the WTO – or of playing off the interests of multiple states to secure their objectives (Jawara and Kwa 2004). The EU operates a common commercial policy and thus negotiates as a single actor at the WTO, concluding shared trade agreements with third parties on behalf of its member states. Trade agreements concluded by the EU and the USA with (economically) smaller states tend to be structured by, and reflect the interests of, those larger economies since smaller economies will be more dependent on access to the European or American markets than vice versa.

The past decade has seen the emergence of what have been dubbed 'mega-regional' trade agreements. One of the best known of these is the Comprehensive and Progressive Trans-Pacific Partnership Agreement (CPTPP), formerly known as the Trans-Pacific Partnership Agreement (TPP) concluded between 11 states in the Pacific region. The USA withdrew from the TPP in 2017, leading to the removal of 22 clauses initially included to satisfy the United States Trade Representative (USTR), the government agency that negotiates international trade agreements on behalf of the US and changes to the ratification mechanisms to allow the renamed CPTPP agreement to come into effect without participation of the USA. In a surprise to geographers, the United Kingdom formally applied to join the CPTPP on 1 February 2021. A similarly ambitious agreement between the EU and the USA – the Trans-Atlantic Trade and Investment Partnership (TTIP) – had been negotiated under the Presidency of Barack Obama but could not be concluded before the end of his second term in January 2017 and the negotiations were frozen by his successor. Such an agreement between the two largest economic blocks would have had significant implications for the global trade regime and for their relations with the world's third economic superpower, China.

BRTIAs have clear implications for health given the propensity they have to liberalize trade beyond the baseline conditions set out in the WTO system. Consequently, many of the arguments about product safety, service regulation and market access for global corporations (including the producers and marketers of harmful products such as tobacco, alcohol and processed food) discussed above are relevant also to debates around BRTIAs (see also Chapter 11). Perhaps the most significant component of these agreements, however, are the extremely robust ISDS mechanisms, which have proven to be a source of significant controversy. These differ from the WTO dispute resolution processes in a number of ways that tilt the balance of power away from sovereign states to the commercial sector. They are held in private with limited transparency and oversight and there is no mechanism to appeal. Perhaps most crucially, these agreements allow private corporations to bring cases against state parties for infringing the protections they enjoy as investors. While in the WTO only other member states could bring such actions – and at times states may be prepared to initiate dispute in the interests of a specific company or sector – under the ISDS provisions within many BRTIAs, corporations and private investors can bring legal actions directly against government (see Box 13.1).

Box 13.1   Trade challenges to Australia's tobacco packaging

In 2012 Australia became the first country in the world to pass laws to ban the branding of cigarette packets. Under the *Tobacco Plain Packaging Act (2011)*, cigarettes must be sold in standardized packs in a uniform colour, size, shape and texture and featuring large graphic health warnings. This closed off one of the last avenues for tobacco branding and marketing activity and was vehemently opposed by the tobacco industry. Various companies launched unsuccessful domestic legal challenges to the measures, citing violations of the Australian constitution (Liberman 2013). At the same time, dispute procedures were initiated against the Australian government at the WTO by Ukraine on the grounds that it violated the country's commitments under TRIPs, GATT and TBT. Ukraine was subsequently joined by the Dominican Republic, Honduras, Cuba and Indonesia as disputing parties, with British American Tobacco and Philip Morris International paying some states' legal expenses (Chapman and Freeman 2013). A WTO panel ruled in favour of Australia in 2018, by which time Ukraine had withdrawn from the case. An appeal was taken forwards by Honduras and the Dominican Republic with the Appellate Body finally settling the case in favour of the Australian government in June 2020.

In parallel with these challenges, Hong-Kong based Philip Morris Asia (PMA), the owner of Philip Morris International's (PMI) Australian subsidiary, initiated investor dispute processes against Australia under the Australia–Hong Kong Bilateral Investment Treaty (AHKBIT). In December 2015 the Permanent Court of Arbitration announced that it had rejected Phillip Morris' claim under the AHKBIT on the grounds that PM Asia only acquired its shareholding in PM's Australian undertaking after the announcement of the proposed legislation to introduce plain packaging (Chapman and Freeman 2013). This undermined any claims by PMA to have suffered materially from the decision, and that it had reasonable or legitimate expectations of a different regulatory environment at the time of investing in the country. The ruling though provides only partial reassurance to public health campaigners since the case was rejected on procedural grounds. The substantive point of law – whether tobacco control measures such as generic packaging contravene the tenets of BRTIAs such as this – remains to be tested. Consequently, legal challenges under ISDS clauses are an avenue that TTCs may continue to exploit. In the meantime, the mere threat of such actions may continue to have a 'chilling effect' on governments elsewhere when they see the difficulties faced even by a high-income country such as Australia (see Côté 2014).

As with the related WTO dispute, PMA's case centred on the importance of branding to cigarette companies. It claims the Australian law (1) is disproportionate and unnecessary in order to guarantee public health in an environment in which there are already significant tobacco control policies in place; (2) enacts protectionist measures that fail to guarantee fair and equitable treatment of non-domestic producers; (3) deprives it of its intellectual property rights and represents a form of indirect expropriation for which compensation is due; and (4) undermines the legitimate expectations that investors would have of the business environment in which they would operate, despite the long history of progressively more stringent tobacco control policies introduced in Australia (Voon and Mitchell 2012; Liberman et al. 2012; Jarman 2015).

The cost to the Australian taxpayers of defending its case against PMA (excluding the case at the WTO) was estimated at almost AUS\$40 million (US\$31.9; £22.5 million), possibly rising to AUS\$50 million. Although the arbitration panel ruled in March 2017 that these costs should be met by PMA, costs are not awarded automatically against the unsuccessful plaintiff. These are significant sums even for high-income countries to absorb and represent a diversion of resources, which could be used for front-line health services. Consequently, this serves as a deterrent to other countries – particularly those with limited resources – to follow suit, especially when uncertainty remains about the compatibility of these policies with other BRTIAs and the recoverability of litigation costs. A similar case of ISDS use by PMI occurred in response to cigarette packet warning labels introduced in Uruguay, highlighting that this is an established industry tactic (see Hawkins and Holden 2016; Hawkins et al. 2018).

The potential for private actors to sue governments via ISDS mechanisms has resulted in a raft of cases brought by some of the world's largest and most powerful corporations against states to oppose progressive environmental and social policies including those designed specifically to protect public health (see Eberhardt and Olivet 2012; Verheecke et al. 2019). Such cases can lead to significant financial awards against governments found to be in breach of their obligations leading even the world's wealthiest countries to change policies. The threat of legal action and the time and costs of fighting such cases even before the judgment can lead government to self-censor, declining to bring forwards policies opposed by powerful vested interests (Hawkins and Holden 2016). Even where states can be confident they will win cases (and avoid awards of compensation against them), the financial costs and human resources needed just to defend such cases are prohibitive for many states and divert the limited resources at their disposal away from essential health services.

The emergence of such cases has led to calls from anti-smoking groups for a 'carve out' of tobacco from the ISDS measures in such agreements. This was partially successful with the CPTPP, with parties to the agreement able to opt in to a non-compulsory tobacco carve out (a mechanism that became dubbed a tobacco 'carve in') (Schram et al. 2019). While this represents progress against corporate interests using trade to undermine health, it remains limited to a very specific area of trade and health policy. This has led campaigners to advocate instead for a more general public health carve out from future agreements, which would include other areas such as alcohol, food and nutrition policy as a way of addressing the global obesity pandemic and the associated rise in non-communicable diseases, a looming crisis for LMICs.

✎ Activity 13.3

Think of some examples of policy proposal or regulations designed to protect public health, which could potentially be subject to legal challenges by companies under BRTIA ISDS clauses. When thinking about this take a broad interpretation of health and the structural determinants of this at the population level such as environmental degradation as well as issues such as tobacco control discussed above.

Feedback

There have been a number of ISDS cases brought against high-income as well as LMIC governments, which have led to changes in policy by those governments or the award of compensation against them. This includes, for example, cases brought against countries like Germany following its decision to cease production of nuclear-generated electricity on environmental and health security grounds. What are far harder to document are the examples of the 'chilling effect' that such cases have on governments who may decide not even to bring forward potentially controversial measures for fear of being subject to expensive and time-consuming legal cases. In reviewing your responses consult the analysis of previous ISDS cases by Eberhardt and Olivet (2012) and Verheecke et al. (2019) and compare these to your cases and examples.

Summary

This chapter examined the ways in which trade, and trade agreements are of relevance to global health. This includes the effects of trade on the wealth and health of populations across the globe as well as the effects it has on the regulatory capacity of states domestically and in the global sphere. Recent decades have seen a shift in emphasis in global trade from a focus exclusively on goods trade to an increasing exchange in cross-border service provision. Similarly, trade agreements have begun to focus increasingly on non-tariff barriers such as regulatory standards and 'behind-the-borders' measures. The multilateral trade regime, with the WTO at its apex has been supplemented by an increasing proliferation of BRTIAs. This has created further grounds for dispute processes to be initiated by states and companies which may restrict the regulatory space for national governments seeking to protect health. Consequently, it is impossible to understand the dynamics of global health without an understanding of the direct and indirect ways in which heath and healthcare are affected by trade.

References

Chapman, S. and Freeman, B. (2013) *Removing the Emperor's Clothes: Australia and Tobacco Plain Packaging.* Sydney: Sydney University Press.

Correa, C. (2004) *Implementation of the WTO General Council Decision on Para 6 of the Doha Declaration on the TRIPS Agreement and Public Health.* EDM Series No. 16. Geneva: World Health Organization.

Côté, C. (2014) *A Chilling Effect? The Impact of International Investment Agreements on National Regulatory Autonomy in the Areas of Health, Safety and the Environment.* The London School of Economics and Political Science (LSE). Available at: http://etheses.lse.ac.uk/897/8/Cote_A_Chilling_%20 Effect.pdf (accessed 12 June 2021).

De Benedictis, L. and Taglioni, D. (2011) The gravity model in international trade, in L. De Benedictis and D. Taglioni (eds) *The Trade Impact of European Union Preferential Policies*. Berlin/ Heidelberg: Springer.

Eberhardt, P. and Olivet, C. (2012) *Profiting from Injustice: How Law Firms, Arbitrators and Financiers Are Fuelling an Investment Arbitration Boom*. Brussels: Corporate Europe Observatory. Available at: http://corporateeurope.org/sites/default/files/publications/profiting-from-injustice.pdf (accessed 12 June 2021).

Gleeson, D., Lexchin, J., Labonté, R. et al. (2019) Analyzing the impact of trade and investment agreements on pharmaceutical policy: provisions, pathways and potential impacts, *Global Health*, 15(78). Available at: https://doi.org/10.1186/s12992-019-0518-2.

Hawkins, B. and Holden, C. (2016) A corporate veto on health policy? Global constitutionalism and investor-state dispute settlement, *Journal of Health Politics, Policy and Law*, 41(5): 969–995.

Hawkins, B., Holden, C. and MacKinder, S. (2018) A multi-level, multi-jurisdictional strategy: transnational tobacco companies' attempts to obstruct tobacco packaging restrictions, *Global Public Health*, 14(4): 570–583.

Jarman, H. (2015) *The Politics of Trade and Tobacco Control*. Basingstoke: Palgrave Macmillan.

Jawara, F. and Kwa, A. (2004) *Behind the Scenes at the WTO: The Real World of International Trade Negotiations*. London: Zed Books.

Lange, S. and Vollmer, S. (2017) The effect of economic development on population health: a review of the empirical evidence, *British Medical Bulletin*, 121(1): 47–60.

Liberman, J. (2013). Plainly constitutional: the upholding of plain tobacco packaging by the High Court of Australia, *American Journal of Law & Medicine*, 39(2–3): 361–381.

Liberman, J., Scollo, M., Freeman, B. et al. (2012) Plain tobacco packaging in Australia: the historical and social context, in T. Voon, A. Mitchell, J. Liberman et al. (eds) *Public Health and Plain Packaging of Cigarettes: Legal Issues*. Cheltenham: Edward Elgar.

Light, D. and Warburton, R. (2011) Demythologizing the high costs of pharmaceutical research, *BioSocieties*, 6(1): 34–50.

Schram, A., Townsend, B., Youde, J. and Friel, S. (2019) Public health over private wealth: rebalancing public and private interests in international trade and investment agreements, *Public Health Research Practice*, 29(3): e2931919.

Sell, S.K. (2003) *Private Power, Public Law: The Globalization of Intellectual Property Rights*. Cambridge: Cambridge University Press.

Sell, S.K. (2007) TRIPS-plus free trade agreements and access to medicines, *Liverpool Law Review*, 28(1): 41–75.

Trading Economics (2013) World: tariff rate, applied, simple mean, all products. Available at: http://globalization.tradingeco-nomics.com/world/tariff-rate-applied-simple-mean-all-products-percent-wb-data.html (accessed 21 June 2021).

Verheecke, L., Eberhardt, P., Olivet, C. et al. (2019) *Red Carpet Courts*. Brussels/Amsterdam: Friends of the Earth Europe and International, The Transparency Institute & Corporate Europe Observatory. Available at: https://corporateeurope.org/sites/default/files/2020-04/Red%20Carpet%20 Courts.pdf (accessed 21 May 2021).

Voon, T. and Mitchell, A. (2012). Implications of international investment law for plain tobacco packaging: lessons from the Hong Kong–Australia BIT, in T. Voon, A. Mitchell, J. Liberman et al. (eds) *Public Health and Plain Packaging of Cigarettes: Legal Issues*. Cheltenham: Edward Elgar.

Conclusions

A brave new world of global health

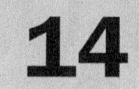

14

Carolyn Stephens, Marco Liverani and Benjamin Hawkins

Overview

This chapter provides a critical reflection on the discussion of globalization, global health and global health governance in this volume. It begins by examining the learning from the book about the highly contested term 'globalization' and identifies the key themes and ideas that run through the preceding chapters. The chapter concludes by placing these reflections in a longer-term perspective, examining the key developments in global health and the critical lessons we have learned from these since the publication of the first edition of this book in 2005.

Learning objectives

After working through this chapter, you will be able to:

- Critically assess the concepts of globalization, governance and global health governance discussed in this book.
- Recognize how the overall themes of this book come together to deepen understanding of globalization and its impact on global health.
- Reflect on the ways in which processes of globalization are of relevance to historical and contemporary issues and debates in global health.

Key terms

Globalization: A set of processes, facilitated by technological developments, leading to greater economic, political, cultural and environmental interconnectedness across the globe.

Global health: A field of research, scholarship, policy and practice focused on health issues where the determinants or outcomes are not contained by the territorial boundaries of states, and thus may be beyond the capacity of individual countries to address them through domestic institutions alone.

> **Governance:**   A series of arrangements consisting of various norms, rules
> and institutional structures through which an area of economic activity,
> public policy or social interaction is regulated and administered by a range
> of public and private actors.
>
> **Global health governance:**   The shifting array of institutions, structures,
> mechanisms and actors through which issues in the arena of global health
> are identified and addressed and through which policy responses are
> decided and implemented.

Revisiting the themes of globalization and health covered in this book

The key terms identified above are the same as those in Chapter 1 since
these concepts provide the conceptual focus of the book as a whole. The
concept of 'globalization' is explored throughout this volume, including
analysis of the debates around this term and reflection on its different
aspects and definitions (e.g. Khondker 2005; Achilles et al. 2018; Bishop
and Payne 2021). It should be noted again that the term globalization is
highly contested, and its precise meaning is a source of constant debate
(e.g. James and Steger 2014).

In examining globalization, the book engaged with the major upstream
processes in the economy, in our social conditions and in the environment,
all of which are key determinants of population health. This book is divided
into three parts and a conclusion: (1) Contextualizing global health; (2) Critical issues in global health; (3) Global health governance; and finally, the
book concludes with this chapter.

Part 1 of the book explored key concepts and critical debates around the
impact of globalization on global health and global health policies. It introduced economic and social change and explored the emergence of global
health governance. Part 1 also sought to place current processes within
their longer-term historical perspective and reflected on the impact of this
history on the current distribution of power within processes of globalization. In particular, it discussed the history of colonial power and its impact
on global health and the evolution of the post-colonial global health movement. Part 2 examined contemporary issues in global health, including
both infectious and non-communicable diseases, and explored their links
to these processes of globalization. It explored the challenges of global
environmental change and the links of global health to debates around
global security. Part 3 identified the main global governance responses to
these issues and the processes and institutional structures which have
emerged to address these. It examined key actors including commercial
actors, non-state actors and bilateral and multilateral actors, and the

issues of global trade and health. Lastly, this chapter concludes the book. Below is a summary of the key messages from each chapter of the book.

Part 1 Contextualizing global health

Chapter 1 discussed the key conceptual challenges of globalization and outlined some of the key characteristics of the changes that this process encompasses. It presented different definitions of globalization and a framework for examining three dimensions of global change: the spatial, temporal and cognitive (Lee 2003).

Chapter 2 identified the key processes and development within the global economy and their relevance for global health, placing the current status of economic globalization within its recent historical context. It identified three key economic trends in recent decades that have shaped the global economy today: increasing international trade, financial globalization and foreign direct investment. These factors have led to the emergence of, and been facilitated by, the creation of global and regional institutions and structures that form the basis of the current system of global economic governance. The chapter discussed the emergence of transnational corporations and business entities that exert significant economic and political power, and whose activities present a significant governance challenge. Developments in the global economy have had a significant impact on levels of global wealth and inequality both between and within states, with significant implications for population health.

Chapter 3 explored the links between globalization and global social changes, and the impact of these on the social determinants of health. It introduced the ideas of shifting demographic and socio-political conditions, and the ideas of the global village and global citizen. It introduced the shifts in norms and values and in the ways in which we communicate and relate to each other. The chapter developed the ideas and concepts of social change that help us to understand the underlying social drivers of some of the shifts in health risks that the following chapters explore.

Chapter 4 explored the history of international and global cooperative efforts to respond to transborder health challenges and sketched some aspects of the historical foundations of contemporary global health governance. The chapter introduced two key themes in these early efforts for transborder cooperation on issues of population health. It argued that some of the patterns of engagement and activity – such as those exhibited in regional cooperation – were consensual, cooperative and driven by common interests among equal partners. It presented evidence that other patterns of engagement, however, were oppressive, intrusive and premised on racist assumptions about the inferiority of indigenous populations. The chapter argued that the politics of colonial extraction and oppression have had a profound influence on shaping the field of global health governance, as well as the ways health priorities are set and health initiatives delivered.

Part 2 Critical issues in global health

Chapter 5 examined the links between globalization and infectious diseases. In the first part, key drivers of disease emergence and transmission were discussed, including increasing human mobility, changes in food production systems and economic inequalities. The second part of the chapter connected with themes explored in Chapter 4, extending the discussion of international cooperation for infectious disease control from early developments in the nineteenth century to the present framework of global disease surveillance. Finally, in the concluding part it was argued that globalization has increased infectious disease risk through complex and multi-dimensional processes but has also encouraged the emergence of new institutions and cooperative arrangements to address these threats.

Chapter 6 examined non-communicable diseases (NCDs) as a global health challenge identifying both behavioural and structural approaches to understanding their incidence and the appropriate policy responses for addressing them. Key risk factors for NCDs – including the consumption of tobacco, alcohol and hyper-processed foods; environmental degradation; and structural changes to the global health economy – have been exacerbated by processes of globalization. This includes the removal of trade barriers, which has led to increased cross-border movements of goods and people, with implications for pollution and air quality, and increased market access to health-harming products heavily promoted by transnational corporations including increasingly in low- and middle-income settings. The global nature of environmental degradations and the transnational nature of the key actors driving the NCD pandemic has led to a proliferation of global agreements designed to address these conditions and their causes. However, these agreements face the challenge of all global policy initiatives in that they are often hard to enforce and to hold governments and other actors to account for their activities.

Chapter 7 explored the links of globalization with global environmental changes (GECs). It presented a global conceptual framework linking GECs to human health. It discussed a range of GECs including climate change, biodiversity loss, loss of food-producing ecosystems, destruction of wetlands, oceans and waste. The issue of monitoring GECs was discussed, as were the health risks related to GECs. The impacts of global environmental change are complex and affect the climate, agricultural production, water, biodiversity, oceans and forests, each of which in turn has an impact on health. The chapter also presented a selection of the global agreements aimed at addressing GECs and the global and national actions that attempt to lead us towards a more sustainable future.

Chapter 8 discussed the links between health and security, grounded in a conceptual understanding of security debates in international relations. It presented competing and conflicting views, critical reasoning and perspectives on how security and health interact, how they *ought to* interact and what some possible implications of these interactions might be. There are benefits and drawbacks to conceptualizing health as a security concern. On the one hand, if health is framed as a national security issue, priority attention and resources are easier to mobilize; on the other hand, there are normative and practical concerns with the appropriateness of such framing. Health issues and their profound existential impacts on individuals and communities, however, can be used as a starting point to re-consider how we think about security and security politics. Health security politics can lead the conceptualizing of security away from exceptional, antagonistic state-level politics and the mobilization of military resources, towards cooperative, empowering, human-centred, transnational efforts to protect human life.

Part 3 Global health governance

Chapter 9 focussed on the role of the state as an actor in global health, differentiating between the internal function of the state (in domestic politics) and its external function (in international affairs). The ability of states to make and enforce laws at the national level stands in contrast to the state of anarchy it faces at the global level and the need for states to come together to form alliances and institutions to manage interdependencies with other states and tackle problems of common concern. Recent decades have seen the emergence of other important actors in global politics including TNCs and international NGOs within an increasingly global civil society. While these have played an important role in things like global health partnerships (GHPs), states remain the predominant and most important actors in global health governance and global politics more generally, responsible for the vast majority of global health funding and the implementation of policies on the ground.

Chapter 10 focused on one of the principal ways in which states manage their relationships and seek common action at the global level: via bilateral, regional and multilateral agreements and structures. While many of these agreements focus on economic governance (with implications for global health), other forms of engagement, particularly at the regional level, have taken the form of far deeper and wide-ranging forms of integration, the most obvious example of which is the EU. At the global level, economic organizations such as the WTO are also relevant to global health, not least in terms of their intellectual property regime and the implications of trade for health. However, WHO and the UN system (e.g. UNAIDS, UNDP, UNHCR, UNICEF, UNHCR) are the multilateral bodies of most direct relevance for health.

Chapter 11 focused on the commercial sector and, in particular, the relevance of TNCs for global health. It argued that corporations are simply too large and economically important to ignore, while their transnational nature means they pose a challenge for governments seeking to regulate their activities. Some companies are engaged directly or through third party bodies in the delivery of health services and medical technologies. At the same time, other sectors are key vectors of disease, with the tobacco, alcohol and processed food sectors producing products which are implicated in the aetiology of a range of chronic diseases of increasing importance to the global burden of disease. These companies aggressively market their products across the globe, resisting regulation and health protecting policies that undermine their business models, including the use of international trade and investment agreements to challenge unfavoured policies. This in turn has implications for democratic oversight and the ability of governments to regulate effectively in the name of public health.

Chapter 12 explored the diversity of civil society organizations (CSOs), philanthropic foundations and global health partnerships and initiatives that have emerged as key actors in contemporary global health. It assessed the increasing significance of these 'new' actors in decision-making at the global level. The chapter explored some key challenges emerging from this proliferation of global health actors: problems of coordinating their increasing numbers, problems of CSOs and foundations maintaining accountability and legitimacy, and the imbalances between large northern and small southern CSOs in terms of their influence on global health decisions.

Chapter 13 examined the international trade regime and its implications for health. Recent decades have seen increasing levels of inertia in the development of the global multilateral trade regime and the emergence of an ever more complex array of bilateral and regional trade and investment agreements. The process of trade liberalization has significant implications for global health in terms of the increased movement of people, goods and services across borders including patients and healthcare professionals, as well as the remote delivery of health services. Increases in the movement of goods and people may facilitate the spread of communicable diseases and commodities implicated in the increasingly global NCD pandemic.

✏ Activity 14.1

Revisit and reflect on the definitions of globalization discussed in Activity 1.1 in the Introduction. Having concluded the book, has your definition of this concept changed? If so, how? Reflect on what you have learned in working through this book. Has this shifted your thinking?

Feedback

As you will have seen, there are very different definitions of globalization in the research literature, some of which are discussed in this book. You may have initially preferred a definition that emphasized the social aspects of these processes, or have thought more about the definitions that emphasized the trade and economic processes. Now you have read the book you may have changed your view on this.

Converging themes in globalization and health

In order to analyse the themes of this book, we needed to divide issues into chapters in a way that does not reflect the ways in which these actors, processes, structures and themes interact and play out in real-world contexts within global health. This section takes three examples of this: the Covid-19 infectious disease pandemic, its social and economic context and consequences; global environmental change and its impact on different societies and peoples across the world; and the increasing importance of private sector actors in the context of globalization and global health governance.

Covid-19: a mirror of globalization

Covid-19 has been an unprecedented global health emergency in recent history, with profound and far-reaching societal impacts. More than any other public health crisis of our time, the pandemic has pervaded every aspect of our lives with direct or indirect effects on physical and mental health, education, work, leisure, relationships and the environment.

As discussed in Chapter 5, Covid-19 is also an illustration of the multidimensional links between global change and health. Theories about the emergence of the disease abound, but it is clear that changing patterns of human mobility and the increase in international travel contributed to the rapid spread of the virus and its variants worldwide. In addition, Covid-19 has laid bare profound global inequities (Oxfam 2021). While the pandemic has affected every sector of the economy in most countries, the economic pressure has been greater in low-income contexts, where millions of people have been pushed back into poverty and even extreme poverty (Marcos Barba et al. 2020).

On a more positive note, the pandemic has demonstrated that, in a globalized world, resources and technologies can be developed and mobilized at impressive speed and on a scale never seen before. Despite the controversies surrounding the Covid-19 immunization programmes (OECD 2021), it is remarkable that the first Covid-19 vaccines were developed, tested, approved and made available to the public less than one year after the initial disease outbreak, based on data openly shared by Chinese scientists (Ledford 2021). During the pandemic, there have also been many stories of courage, hope and dedication such as the stories of health workers facing higher risk of infection and enduring overnight shifts in overwhelmed health facilities (Mehta et al. 2021). And there have been many stories of solidarity. In Thailand, for example, volunteers launched a 'Pantry of Sharing' initiative, where people could donate non-perishable food items and basic hygiene supplies to others who were in need during the outbreaks (Bangkok Post 2020).

Nonetheless, Covid-19 remains a prominent reminder that our societies can be vulnerable to an extent we could not even imagine, exposing profound inequities within and across countries. In light of this experience, therefore, we should draw important lessons not only to strengthen our pandemic preparedness but also to build the foundations for a more equitable and sustainable economic order. As the recipient of the Nobel Prize in Economics Joseph Stiglitz pointed out, the impact of the pandemic on employment and the labour market has further highlighted that 'the rules governing globalization must do more than just serve corporate interests: workers and the environment have to be protected' (Stiglitz 2020).

Global environmental change: multiple actors and converging priorities

Chapter 7 focused on describing the key GECs occurring globally and looked at some key global agreements to address them. Chapters 2 and 3 looked at the key economic and social trends linked to globalization. Chapter 12 looked at key non-governmental actors involved in global health. When you put these four chapters together, you can start to see the ways in which global economic and social trends – particularly economic trends in increased production and social trends in increased consumption – have links with global environmental changes (UNDP 2020). This is having catastrophic effects on the planet. In the first edition of this textbook, Professor Tony McMichael predicted likely future effects of climate changes on a range of environmental conditions and human health impacts (McMichael 2005). Just over 15 years later, in our third edition of this textbook, IPCC scientists now know that 'human-induced climate change is already affecting many weather and climate extremes in every region across the globe. Evidence of observed changes in extremes such as heatwaves, heavy precipitation, droughts, and tropical cyclones, and, in particular, their attribution to human influence, has strengthened since the Fifth Assessment Report' (IPCC 2021).

The urgency of the need to address global environmental changes is reflected in actions across governments, the private sector and civil society. For example, looking at the commercial sector and the energy sector, in 2005 there was still debate around the human influence on climate changes and strong resistance to change from parts of the commercial sector. In 2021, there are a number of examples of actions by the actors in the sector that start to bring it in line with goals of sustainable development. Although many analysts are sceptical about the role and responsibility of commercial actors in GECs, there is no doubt that their actions are highly important – either for good or bad. For example, IPIECA (originally the International Petroleum Industry Environmental Conservation Association) is now the global oil and gas industry association for environmental and social issues, including all the major corporate actors in the oil and gas sectors. IPIECA has a number of global roles. It has worked with the United

Nations Development Programme (UNDP) and the International Finance Corporation (IFC) to develop an atlas of the implications of the UN Sustainable Development Goals for the oil and gas industry and how the industry can most effectively contribute to the achievement of the SDGs (IFC/IPIECA/UNDP 2017). There are also long standing interventions: on a practical and critical issue – related to oil spills and marine pollution, IPIECA has been working since 1996 with the International Maritime Organization (IMO) (the UN agency responsible for the safety and security of shipping and the prevention of marine pollution by shipping) to establish oil spill preparedness and response in some of the most important ecosystems internationally (Coolbaugh et al. 2014).

The other key set of actors working on GECs (discussed in Chapter 12) are the non-governmental actors – of which there are now thousands, ranging from local civil society groups organized around local environmental problems, to non-governmental organizations accredited by the United Nations to participate at a global level. These civil society actors bring a critical voice to the table on GECs – including monitoring commercial actors and bringing their actions to global attention. Global actors include long standing high-profile international environmental non-governmental organizations (IENGOs) such as direct-action non-governmental actor Greenpeace, founded in 1971 and now present in over 40 countries, and Friends of the Earth International (FOEI), also started in 1971 by sister organizations from France, Sweden, England and the USA. FOEI is now a federation of 73 member organizations, of which approximately half are called 'Friends of the Earth' in native languages of the country members, and other members use different names. It is important to note the continuing repercussions of past colonial and economic power imbalances between ENGOs. Importantly, these issues of power between environmental NGOs are increasingly highlighted and challenged. An analysis in 2020 of 679 global environmental NGOs (ENGOs) found that there were significant human and financial resource disparities between ENGOs in the Global North versus Global South and challenged the sector to change (Partelow et al. 2020).

In terms of the importance of civil society actors in the global policy arena, there is significant evidence that IENGOs have been increasingly influential and important at a global level in support of climate change agreements such as the Paris Agreement (Allan and Hadden 2017). Again, analysts are concerned that there is inequality in both representation and perspective between northern and southern NGOs represented in international climate change negotiations. This is particularly important because ENGOs from the Global North form the vast majority of NGOs taking part in negotiations, and the perspective and agendas of these two sets of ENGOs are often very different – with southern NGOs often highlighting global environmental injustice (Gereke and Brühl 2019).

As GECs accelerate, their impact will be felt globally but unevenly. GECs are already disproportionately negatively affecting poorer nations and poorer peoples, and this is likely to continue. Global inequities in decision-making power between nation states and between other actors will affect the direction and focus of global policy. The reality of the uneven responsibility for GECs already creates tensions globally, and this too is likely to continue. Challenges to this power structure are now well articulated through critical academic reflection and within state and non-state actor debates. This may produce change in the future. However these power relations evolve, there is now little doubt that global collective action is the only way really to deal with GECs.

The 'commercialization' of global health in the context of globalization

As noted above, recent decades have seen profound changes in the structure of the global economy, which were summarized in Chapter 2. One aspect of this has been the consolidation of ownership within sectors – including health-harming industries such as the tobacco and alcohol sectors (Hawkins et al. 2018) – which has seen the emergence of powerful transnational corporations that dominate the markets in which they are active. As a result of processes of trade liberalization, discussed in Chapter 13, these companies are often active across the globe and are increasingly seeking opportunities for growth in LMICs. The entry of the companies into such markets is often associated with an increase in consumption of their products due to greater competition, increased marketing spend and price reductions (Gleeson and Labonté 2020). This has implications for public health in contexts where health systems and public finances are ill equipped to deal with the dual burden of increasing NCD morbidity emerging alongside ongoing pressures of infectious disease control. At the same time, TNCs are intrinsically involved in the provisions and delivery of health services and treatments (i.e. private hospitals and facilities, medical devices, pharmaceuticals, health insurance).

However, it is perhaps in the area of global health governance that the influence of corporations and other private sector actors is most indicative of wider trends in the ongoing process of globalization. As we saw in Chapter 9, politics in the global sphere is defined by the conditions of anarchy and the absence of an overarching authority to set the rules of the game, enforce agreements and police the behaviour of states and other policy actors. This means states have a disincentive to adhere to international agreements for fear that others will not do likewise and gain an advantage from this (e.g. there may be a perceived economic advantage from breaking the terms of global climate accords to limit carbon outputs). In the context of globalization, states face a further challenge in that many of the companies whose activities they may seek to regulate in order to protect health may have turnover and profits in excess of the GNP and public sector resources of medium-sized and even larger economies. Moreover, their presence in multiple jurisdictions, and their integrated global structures, mean it is extremely difficult for any single government acting in isolation to hold them to account. For example, attempts to introduce taxes on corporate profits – to fund health services and other public policies – may lead companies to 'relocate' their resources to other 'tax-efficient' settings, meaning that a global response is needed in order to prevent corporate tax avoidance. Such an approach was proposed by the G7 countries at their summit in June 2021, leading to the conclusions of a landmark global agreement on corporate taxation (HM Treasury 2021). This seeks to tie taxation to the location in which corporate profits are generated as opposed to where the most favourable tax rates are applied. While this represents a first step in the direction of policing the affairs of TNCs and ensuring they contribute fairly to the societies in which they generate their profits, it remains limited in its scope to the high-income countries which make up the group. Nonetheless, this represents an important development, which acknowledges the need for collective supranational action to address corporate power and potentially lays the foundations for a more universal approach through other institutional structures.

Another consequence of globalization and the emergence of transnational health policy challenges is the opportunity this affords TNCs – and other civil society actors examined in Chapter 12 – to seek to fill the governance gaps in the global system noted above. The difficulties in establishing binding and enforceable global policy responses, for example in the area of NCD control discussed in Chapter 6, has led policy actors to consider other governance approaches including self- and co-regulatory regimes such as the UN Global Compact discussed in Chapter 11. The challenge of providing solutions to global health problems has led to the emergence of new forms of governance structure. Chapter 12 looked at the role of civil society in global health policy, including philanthropic bodies established with the profits from global corporations (e.g. the Bill and Melinda Gates Foundation), as well as other civil society actors in the formation of global health partnerships. Public–private partnerships and co-regulatory initiatives have been criticized for their ineffectiveness while allowing private sector actors extensive access to global governance actors. In addition, in affording private sector actors a seat at the global governance table it allows them to define themselves as key policy stakeholders and so frame problems and policy solutions in business-friendly ways that can be addressed through partnership based approaches. Despite these criticisms, it can be argued that in the context of globalization, and the conditions of anarchy that undermine the possibility of more robust forms of regulation, that there is no alternative to these forms of collaborative governance arrangement.

Globalization and health – looking at global changes since the first edition

This book is the third edition of the volume first published in 2005 under the title *Global Change and Health* (Lee and Collin 2005). A second edition

(Hanefeld 2015) followed a decade later under the title *Globalization and Health*. The publication of the current text offers the opportunity to reflect on developments in global health, global governance and the wider political economy of globalization in the intervening period. The decreasing intervals between volumes reflects in part the increasing pace of technological, environmental, economic and socio-political change seen in the last 15 years – which has necessitated an almost constant process of reassessment and reappraisal of the contexts under study by academics and other analysts.

This is not to say that events have unfolded in a linear or teleological way. Many developments, which were unforeseeable in 2005, have emerged and revolutionized the way we live our lives, the nature of the health challenges we face and the potential responses to these in ways which simply could not have been predicted in advance. The emergence of social media, for example (and associated advance in the communications technologies that underpin these), has had a seismic and disruptive effect on the way in which information is shared, with implications for the structure of the global economy and society as well as opening new horizons for health diagnostics and treatment. The impacts of GECs globally are already being felt, and people around the world are conscious of the massive challenge this poses to human health and planetary health.

During the Covid-19 pandemic, much of the economy was able to continue in modified forms through online home working and study in ways which would have been impossible at the time of the first volume, allowing effective public health interventions to be implemented with far greater percentages of the global population able to isolate at home for far longer than would have been possible before. As the same time, the new information environment poses a potential health challenge in terms of the way in which misinformation can spread. While the effects of social media on mental health have been an object of concern for some time, the wider effects of social media and the changing information environment as structural determinants of health are only now emerging as key elements of the research agenda in global health.

The global environmental crisis has risen in global profile since the first edition (UNDP 2020). In the 15 years since the first edition there have been two notable shifts. The first is the consensus of scientists around the human responsibility for the global environmental changes the planet is experiencing – with the current era now accepted by the United Nations as the Anthropocene (UNDP 2020). Second is the consensus of governments and much of civil society globally on the need to act, leading to a plethora of actions from community level to the UN (UNDP and University of Oxford 2021). It is clear that the impacts of these GECs are already being felt unevenly, and the responsibility for these GECs is held very unevenly between and within countries. It is highly significant that the UNDP decided in 2020 to update the Human Development Index (HDI) to add a measure of impact of a country's population on the planet – 30 years after the first HDI was launched – to add social aspects of development to measures of human progress (UNDP 2020). It will be interesting to see how countries evolve on this new aspect of the HDI and where this global collection of actions will have taken the planet and global health policy when it is next necessary to update these themes.

The change in title between the first and second editions symbolized the importance of globalization as an analytical concept and the underlying processes of change within global society which it attempts to capture. At the time at which the second volume emerged, many commentators would have seen globalization as an inexorable logic moving towards ever closer economic and political forms of interconnection and interdependence. Events in recent years have called this into question. What we are faced with today is a recognition that globalization is not just an uneven process – touching the lives of different peoples across the globe in different ways and to different extents – but proceeds at an uneven pace and may not be unidirectional. The election of politicians in countries like the US and Brazil on explicitly anti-globalist agendas as well as the newly re-assertive nationalism evident in other countries across the globe pose a challenge to the logic of globalization and for the collective global action on climate change and other common challenges.

While much has changed, there are many constants evident across the volumes. The nation state, for instance, remains a key global health actor and global policy responses remain constrained by the same conditions of possibility for collective political action at the global sphere. Other long-standing actors – civil society and corporations – have assumed new or evolving roles. The skewed burden of infectious diseases in LMICs continues to endure but has been matched by the increasing prevalence of NCDs in increasing areas of the globe. GECs will only increase in importance both in terms of impacts and as global policy priorities. Perhaps the key lesson to be learned from the series of these volumes is that the area of global health is continually evolving and while some of the issues we will face in the future will continue along well-established trajectories, many of the key challenges we face may yet be unknown or may come to affect us in ways which are not yet apparent.

Summary

This final chapter has looked at the overall themes that we have addressed in this book. We have summarized the key points from each of the chapters. We have looked at how strands of analysis in different chapters work together to explain key themes and have reflected on the changes that we have seen since the first edition of this book. We hope that you will continue this reflection.

References

Achilles, M., Kunakhovich, K. and Shea, N. (2018) Nationalism, nativism, and the revolt against globalization, *Europe Now.* Council for European Studies. Available at: https://globalization.europenow-journal.org/2018/01/31/nationalism-nativism-and-the-revolt-against-globalization/ (accessed 21 June 2021).

Allan, J. and Hadden, J. (2017) Exploring the framing power of NGOs in global climate politics, *Environmental Politics*, 26:4, 600–620. DOI: 10.1080/09644016.2017.1319017.

Bangkok Post (2020) 'Pantries of sharing' fan out nationwide. 12 May 2020. Available at: https://globalization.bangkokpost.com/thailand/general/1916380/pantries-of-sharing-fan-out-nationwide.

Bishop, M. and Payne, A. (2021) The political economies of different globalizations: theorizing reglobalization, *Globalizations*, 18(1): 1–21. DOI: 10.1080/14747731.2020.1779963.

Coolbaugh, T., Bonneville, E., Depraz, S. et al. (2014) The IMO/IPIECA Global Initiative: expanding government and industry cooperation into new regions. International Oil Spill Conference Proceedings, 2014(1): 1342–1352. Available at: https://doi.org/10.7901/2169-3358-2014.1.1342.

Gereke, M. and Brühl, T. (2019) Unpacking the unequal representation of Northern and Southern NGOs in international climate change politics, *Third World Quarterly*, 40(5): 870–889. DOI: 10.1080/01436597.2019.1596023.

Gleeson, D. and Labonté, R. (2020) *Trade Agreements and Public Health*. Singapore: Springer.

Hanefeld, J. (2015) *Globalization and Health*. Maidenhead: Open University Press.

Hawkins, B., Holden, C., Eckhardt, J. et al. (2018) Reassessing policy paradigms: a comparison of the global tobacco and alcohol industries, *Global Public Health*, 13(1): 1–19.

HM Treasury (2021) G7 Finance ministers agree historic global tax agreement. Available at: https://globalization.gov.uk/government/news/g7-finance-ministers-agree-historic-global-tax-agreement (accessed 13 July 2021).

IFC/IPIECA/UNDP (2017) *Mapping the Oil and Gas Industry to the SDGs: An Atlas.* Available at: https://globalization.undp.org/publications/mapping-oil-and-gas-industry-sdgs-atlas (accessed 25 June 2021).

IPCC (2021) Climate Change 2021: The Physical Science Basis. Contribution of Working Group I to the Sixth Assessment Report of the Intergovernmental Panel on Climate Change [V. Masson-Delmotte, P. Zhai, A. Pirani et al. (eds.)]. Cambridge: Cambridge University Press. In press.

James, P. and Steger, M. (2014) A genealogy of 'globalization': the career of a concept, *Globalizations*, 11(4): 417–434. DOI: 10.1080/14747731.2014.951186.

Khondker, H. (2005) Globalization to glocalisation: a conceptual exploration, *Intellectual Discourse*, 13(2). Available at: https://journals.iium.edu.my/intdiscourse/index.php/id/article/view/109 (accessed 21 June 2021)

Ledford, H. (2021) Six months of COVID vaccines: what 1.7 billion doses have taught scientists, *Nature*, 594(7862): 164–167. DOI: 10.1038/d41586-021-01505-x.

Lee, K. (2003) *Globalization and Health: An Introduction.* London: Palgrave Macmillan.

Lee, K. and Collin, J. (eds) (2005) *Global Change and Health*. Buckingham: Open University Press.

Marcos Barba, L., van Regenmortel, H. and Ehmke, E. (2020) *Shelter from the Storm. The Global Need for Universal Social Protection in Times of COVID-19*. Oxford: Oxfam International.

Mehta, S., Machado, F., Kwizera, A. et al. (2021) Covid-19: a heavy toll on health-care workers, *Lancet Respiratory Medicine*, 9(3): 226–228. DOI: 10.1016/S2213-2600(21)00068-0.

McMichael, A. (2005) Global environmental changes, climate change and human health, in K. Lee and J. Collin (eds) *Global Change and Health*. Buckingham: Open University Press.

OECD (2021) *Enhancing Public Trust in Covid-19 Vaccination: The Role of Governments, OECD Policy Responses to Coronavirus (Covid-19)*. Paris: OECD Publishing. Available at: https://doi.org/10.1787/eae0ec5a-en.

Oxfam (2021) *The Inequality Virus. Bringing Together a World Torn Apart by Coronavirus Through a Fair, Just and Sustainable Economy*. Oxford: Oxfam International. Available at: https://oxfam.app.box.com/s/m7lab231vgyee3hti2qjgu8qvc6o9wd1/file/764213341297 (accessed 12 July 2021).

Partelow, S., Winkler, K.J. and Thaler, G.M. (2020) Environmental non-governmental organizations and global environmental discourse, *PLoS ONE*, 15(5): e0232945. DOI: 10.1371/journal.pone.0232945.

Stiglitz, J. (2020) Conquering the great divide, *Finance & Development*, Fall 2020 issue. Washington, DC: The International Monetary Fund. Available at: https://globalization.imf.org/external/pubs/ft/fandd/2020/09/COVID19-and-global-inequality-joseph-stiglitz.htm (accessed 12 July 2021).

UNDP (2020) *Human Development Report 2020. The Next Frontier: Human Development and the Anthropocene*. United Nations Development Programme. Available at: http://hdr.undp.org/sites/default/files/hdr2020.pdf (accessed 18 May 2021).

WHO, UN and UNICEF et al. (2020) Managing the Covid-19 infodemic: promoting healthy behaviours and mitigating the harm from misinformation and disinformation. Joint statement by WHO, UN, UNICEF, UNDP, UNESCO, UNAIDS, ITU, UN Global Pulse, and IFRC. Available at: https://globalization.who.int/news/item/23-09-2020-managing-the-Covid-19-infodemic-promoting-healthy-behaviours-and-mitigating-the-harm-from-misinformation-and-disinformation (accessed 12 June 2021).

Index

01 14

Printed and bound by CPI Group (UK) Ltd, Croydon, CR0 4YY

14/11/2024

01788858-0009